Patient Outcomes in Medical-Surgical Nursing

Nancy H. Camp, RN,C, MSN
Director of Education
Mercy Haverford Hospital
Haverford, Pennsylvania

Patricia Iyer, RN, MSN, CNA
President
Patricia Iyer Associates
Stockton, New Jersey

Springhouse Corporation
Springhouse, Pennsylvania

Staff

EXECUTIVE DIRECTOR, EDITORIAL
Stanley Loeb

SENIOR PUBLISHER, TRADE AND TEXTBOOKS
Minnie B. Rose, RN, BSN, MEd

ART DIRECTOR
John Hubbard

CLINICAL EDITOR
Patricia Kardish Fischer, RN, BSN

SENIOR EDITOR
Kathy Goldberg

ASSOCIATE ACQUISITIONS EDITOR
Caroline Lemoine

COPY EDITORS
Debra Davis, Barbara Hodgson, Charles Peitz

DESIGNERS
Stephanie Peters (Associate Art Director), Cindy Marczuk

EDITORIAL ASSISTANT
Louise Quinn

MANUFACTURING
Deborah Meiris (director), Anna Brindisi, Kate Davis, T.A. Landis

Printed in the United States of America. For information, write Springhouse Corporation, 1111 Bethlehem Pike, P.O. Box 908, Springhouse, PA 19477-0908.

PTOUTMS-01109

A member of the Reed Elsevier plc group

Library of Congress Cataloging-in-Publication Data
Camp, Nancy Hand.
Patient outcomes in medical-surgical nursing/ Nancy H. Camp, Patricia Iyer.
p. cm.
Includes bibliographical references and index.
1. Nursing. 2. Surgical nursing. 3. Outcome assessment (Medical care) 4. Nursing diagnosis. I. Iyer, Patricia W. II. Title.
[DNLM: 1. Nursing diagnosis–methods. 2. Surgical Nursing–methods. 3. Outcome and Process Assessment (Health Care) WY 161 C186p 1994]
RT41.C277 1994
610.73–dc20
DNLM/DLC
94-27904
ISBN 0-87434-701-7 CIP

Table of Contents

Neurologic System

Endocrine System

Genitourinary System

Reproductive System

Musculoskeletal and Integumentary Systems

Hematologic and Immunologic Systems

Psychiatric Disorders

Appendices

Acknowledgments and Dedication

The author wishes to acknowledge the valuable contributions of the clinical reviewer, Carrie A. McCoy, RN, MSN, CEN, Associate Professor of Nursing, Northern Kentucky University, and the Series Editor, Patricia Iyer, RN, MSN.

Dedication

To my husband, John Camp,
and my son, Matthew Camp
To my parents,
and
To the memory of my brother, Bill

Preface

Patient Outcomes in Medical-Surgical Nursing is designed to be a reference for nurses interested in providing quality care with a focus on outcomes. Knowledge of outcomes is critical in the current health care environment. Outcomes serve as the framework for providing efficient, effective care within the prescribed length of stay.

Traditional care plan books commonly emphasize the nursing diagnosis, interventions, and rationale for actions. *Patient Outcomes in Medical-Surgical Nursing* stresses the nursing diagnoses, desired patient outcomes, outcome criteria, and selected nursing interventions for a variety of medical diagnoses commonly seen in the acute care medical-surgical setting.

The medical diagnoses are grouped according to body systems and alphabetized for easy reference. Each medical diagnosis presents a variety of NANDA-approved nursing diagnoses associated with that particular medical diagnosis.

The desired patient outcome is formulated as a general statement expressing the positive outcome that the patient and the health care team will work together to achieve. The outcome measurement criteria are the benchmarks used to determine the degree of outcome achievement. Selected nursing interventions are included to assist the nurse in planning care and promoting positive patient outcomes.

The nursing diagnoses address the physical, psychosocial, spiritual, and cognitive needs of the patient and family. Recognizing the key role the family plays in the patient's recovery, the term family is used throughout the text in the broadest sense to describe one's "family of choice"—not just one's family of origin. The expanded use of advanced-practice nurses to deliver primary health care is reflected in the terms used in this text. Instead of referring to the physician, we have used the more generic term of primary health care practitioner or provider. This acknowledges the role of the nurse practitioner in delivering primary health care in an outpatient setting.

Appendices include the most recent list of NANDA-approved nursing diagnoses, a list of the medical diagnoses and associated nursing diagnoses presented in the body of the text, and selected references.

Abdominal aortic aneurysm repair

Surgical replacement, using a graft, of an abdominal aortic aneurysm (localized dilatation and weakening of middle layer of abdominal aortic wall); without surgical repair, aneurysm may rupture and cause death.

NURSING DIAGNOSIS

Anxiety related to effects of impending surgical procedure and postoperative recovery

DESIRED PATIENT OUTCOME

The patient will express tolerance of anxiety about the surgical outcome

Outcome measurement criteria

- ☐ Verbalization of concerns and fears
- ☐ Verbalization of understanding of surgical procedure and postoperative care
- ☐ Relaxed facial expression and posture
- ☐ Demonstration of relaxation techniques to help control anxiety
- ☐ Demonstration of correct techniques for coughing, deep breathing, and splinting the incision

Key interventions

- Assess the patient for physiologic and nonverbal signs of anxiety. Listen for verbal cues indicating increased anxiety.
- Encourage the patient to express concerns and fears.

- Explain preoperative and postoperative care.
- Teach relaxation techniques, such as deep breathing and guided imagery.
- Teach correct techniques for coughing, deep breathing, and splinting. Observe return demonstration.
- Maintain calm environment.

NURSING DIAGNOSIS

High risk for fluid volume deficit related to complications of aneurysm repair

DESIRED PATIENT OUTCOME

The patient will maintain an adequate fluid balance

Outcome measurement criteria

☐ Stable vital signs

☐ Normal skin color and temperature

☐ Serum electrolyte levels within normal ranges

☐ Urine output of at least 30 ml/hour

☐ Absence of signs or symptoms of internal or external hemorrhage

Key interventions

- Provide fluid replacement, as ordered.
- Monitor vital signs every 4 hours.
- Monitor hydration status by assessing mucous membranes, skin turgor, and blood pressure.
- Weigh the patient and document result daily.
- Monitor fluid intake and output, including amounts from all tubes and wound drainage.
- Assess wound and dressing for signs of bleeding at least every 4 hours.

- Assess all drainage for blood.
- Monitor serum electrolyte values daily.

NURSING DIAGNOSIS

High risk for infection related to inflammation secondary to surgical trauma

DESIRED PATIENT OUTCOME

The patient will remain free of infection during the postoperative period

Outcome measurement criteria

- ☐ Oral temperature at or below 99.0° F (37.2° C)
- ☐ White blood cell (WBC) count within normal range
- ☐ Absence of erythema, tenderness, and purulent drainage at incision site
- ☐ Approximation of wound edges
- ☐ Negative wound cultures

Key interventions

- Measure oral temperature at least every 4 hours.
- Monitor WBC count for increases that suggest infection. Report abnormal results to the physician.
- Assess wound for signs of infection during each shift.
- Obtain wound cultures, as ordered, and monitor results.
- Consult the infection control practitioner, as needed.

NURSING DIAGNOSIS

Pain related to inflammation and immobility secondary to surgical tissue trauma

DESIRED PATIENT OUTCOME

The patient will express relief from pain

Outcome measurement criteria

☐ Verbalization of adequate pain relief

☐ Relaxed facial expression and muscle tone

☐ Vital signs within normal ranges

Key interventions

- Assess the patient for signs and symptoms of pain, including increased blood pressure, facial grimaces, splinting, shallow breathing, irritability, and restlessness.
- Explain management of postoperative pain, including meaning of *p.r.n.*
- Instruct the patient to request pain medication before pain becomes severe.
- Discuss use of around-the-clock pain medication schedule with the physician to achieve better pain control.
- Teach the patient correct use of patient-controlled analgesia pump, if applicable.
- Use additional pain control methods, such as relaxation, music, and guided imagery, as adjuncts to medication.
- Monitor and document effectiveness of pain medication.
- Consult the physician and clinical pharmacist if pain management is ineffective.

NURSING DIAGNOSIS

High risk for altered peripheral tissue perfusion related to reduced arterial blood flow

DESIRED PATIENT OUTCOME

The patient will maintain adequate arterial blood flow

Outcome measurement criteria

- ☐ Presence of peripheral pulses
- ☐ Normal skin color and temperature
- ☐ Absence of pain, numbness, or tingling in extremities
- ☐ Urine output of at least 30 ml/hour

Key interventions

- Assess peripheral pulses at least every 4 hours. Document presence and intensity of pulses. Immediately notify the physician of any changes.
- Assess extremities for color, temperature, and capillary refill.
- Monitor fluid intake and output for signs of deteriorating renal function.
- Instruct the patient to report pain, numbness, or tingling in extremities immediately.

Acute myocardial infarction

Ischemia and necrosis of myocardium resulting from interruption of blood supply from coronary arteries to the affected area.

NURSING DIAGNOSIS

Activity intolerance related to imbalance between oxygen supply and demand

DESIRED PATIENT OUTCOME

The patient will tolerate a gradual increase in activity

Outcome measurement criteria

- ☐ Demonstration of ability to perform self-care activities independently
- ☐ Demonstration of ability to ambulate independently
- ☐ Heart rate of 110 beats/minute or lower, or increasing no more than 20 beats/minute over baseline during activity
- ☐ Heart rate returning to normal range within 5 minutes after the patient stops activity
- ☐ Absence of chest pain, diaphoresis, and dyspnea
- ☐ Absence of dizziness and fatigue
- ☐ Absence of cardiac arrhythmias that differ from baseline findings

Key interventions

- Monitor physiologic response to increased activity.
- Teach the patient how to monitor own pulse.
- Provide oxygen, as prescribed.

- Provide adequate rest between activities.
- Instruct the patient to report chest pain, dyspnea, or associated symptoms immediately.
- Explain interrelationships between oxygen supply, oxygen demand, and physical activity.
- Encourage the patient to participate in activities of daily living to tolerance level.
- Refer the patient to outpatient cardiac rehabilitation program, if available.

NURSING DIAGNOSIS

Pain (chest) related to ischemia

DESIRED PATIENT OUTCOME

The patient will experience relief from chest pain

Outcome measurement criteria

- ☐ Absence of chest pain
- ☐ Relaxed facial expression and muscle tone
- ☐ Absence of diaphoresis, nausea, and associated signs and symptoms
- ☐ Vital signs within normal ranges
- ☐ Verbalization of reduction in or relief from pain

Key interventions

- Assess and document the patient's description of chest pain, including quality, location, radiation, duration, and precipitating and alleviating factors.
- Observe for associated signs and symptoms, including cool and clammy skin, diaphoresis, dyspnea, nausea, and vomiting.
- Monitor vital signs during and after pain episodes.

- Administer oxygen, as prescribed.
- Administer pain medication, as prescribed, and document effectiveness.
- Report changes in the patient's status to the physician.

NURSING DIAGNOSIS

Ineffective denial related to perceived threat to health and life-style

DESIRED PATIENT OUTCOME

The patient will discuss the impact of current health status on health and life-style

Outcome measurement criteria

- □ Verbalization of feelings and perceptions of health status
- □ Verbalization of support systems, such as family, friends, and religious institution
- □ Demonstration of effective coping strategies
- □ Relaxed facial expression and posture
- □ Verbalization of intention to modify life-style, if applicable
- □ Verbalization of intention to seek follow-up health care after discharge

Key interventions

- Assess the patient's perception of current health problem.
- Discuss problem-solving techniques the patient has used in past.
- Encourage the patient to verbalize feelings regarding current health problem.

- Provide uninterrupted time with the patient (other than when providing care) to discuss concerns.
- Assist the patient in identifying existing support systems.
- Encourage the patient to use support systems to assist with coping.
- Explain all care and procedures.
- Answer the patient's questions to help reduce anxiety.
- Maintain nonjudgmental approach.
- Assist the patient in developing problem-solving skills.

NURSING DIAGNOSIS

High risk for ineffective management of therapeutic regimen related to denial and knowledge deficit

DESIRED PATIENT OUTCOME

The patient will develop a plan for integrating components of the therapeutic regimen into daily living

Outcome measurement criteria

☐ Verbalization of understanding of preventive health measures, such as stress management, dietary modifications, and exercise

☐ Demonstration of adherence to dietary modifications during hospitalization

☐ Verbalization of willingness to stop smoking, if applicable

☐ Identification of personal risk factors and stressors that may lead to further cardiac problems

☐ Verbalization of names, purposes, dosages, and common adverse effects of prescribed medications

☐ Verbalization of willingness to adhere to prescribed medical regimen after discharge

Key interventions

- Assess the patient's readiness to learn about therapeutic regimen, as demonstrated by asking questions, reading pamphlets, and attending available classes.
- Describe, in simple terms, basic pathophysiology of myocardial infarction and associated symptoms.
- Assist the patient in identifying personal risk factors and stressors.
- Use various means to provide information, including videos, printed materials, and group classes. Include the family in teaching sessions whenever possible.
- Instruct the patient to report chest, back, or jaw pain immediately.
- Discuss role of exercise in reducing weight, blood pressure, and serum lipid levels.
- Consult the dietitian for instructions regarding low-fat, low-sodium diet. Reinforce the dietitian's instructions with the patient.
- Explain relationship between smoking and heart disease.
- Discuss stress management and relaxation as ways to deal with stressors associated with daily living.
- Discuss names, purposes, dosages, and common adverse effects of prescribed medications.
- Describe activity guidelines, such as when to return to work and resume sexual activity and how to modify activity during temperature extremes.
- Refer the patient to outpatient cardiac rehabilitation program, if available.
- Provide list of weight-management groups, smoking-cessation classes, and cardiac support groups, as applicable.

Angina pectoris

Chest pain caused by imbalance between oxygen supply and demand, resulting from transient insufficiency of coronary blood flow (such as from obstruction, spasm, or constriction).

NURSING DIAGNOSIS

Pain (chest) related to imbalance between oxygen supply and demand

DESIRED PATIENT OUTCOME

The patient will experience relief from chest pain

Outcome measurement criteria

- ☐ Verbalization of decrease in pain within 20 minutes of intervention
- ☐ Absence of diaphoresis, nausea, dyspnea, and cool and clammy skin
- ☐ Vital signs within normal ranges
- ☐ Relaxed facial expression and muscle tone

Key interventions

- Assess and document the patient's description of pain, including quality, location, duration, radiation, and precipitating and alleviating factors. Note presence of nausea, dyspnea, diaphoresis, and other associated symptoms.
- Monitor vital signs during and after chest pain episodes.
- Administer antianginal medications, as prescribed. Monitor the patient's vital signs and response to medication.

- Obtain 12-lead electrocardiogram during chest pain episodes.
- Administer oxygen, as prescribed.
- Establish and maintain intravenous (I.V.) access, as ordered, for possible administration of I.V. analgesics.
- Instruct the patient to stop activity when pain arises and to rest until pain subsides.

NURSING DIAGNOSIS

Anxiety related to chest pain episodes

DESIRED PATIENT OUTCOME

The patient will demonstrate abated signs of anxiety

Outcome measurement criteria

☐ Verbalization of concerns and fears

☐ Verbalization of realistic prognosis

☐ Relaxed facial expression and posture

☐ Use of breathing techniques that promote relaxation during anxiety-provoking situations

☐ Demonstration of desire to learn about angina to decrease anxiety

Key interventions

- Assess the patient for signs and symptoms of anxiety, including verbal cues.
- Encourage the patient to verbalize concerns and fears.
- Assist the patient in identifying and describing feelings and sources of anxiety.
- Minimize anxiety-producing events.
- Encourage participation in diversional activities.

- Teach breathing techniques that promote relaxation.
- Encourage the patient to ask questions and gain information about medical condition.
- Provide timely and accurate information. Answer the patient's questions honestly.

NURSING DIAGNOSIS

High risk for altered health maintenance related to the need to modify risk factors

DESIRED PATIENT OUTCOME

The patient and family will verbalize an understanding of the importance of modifying risk factors

Outcome measurement criteria

- ☐ Identification of personal risk factors
- ☐ Verbalization of factors that precipitate chest pain
- ☐ Selection of foods that conform with prescribed dietary modifications
- ☐ Verbalization of willingness to stop smoking, if applicable
- ☐ Discussion of correct use of prescribed medication
- ☐ Demonstration of correct technique for self-administering prescribed sublingual nitrates
- ☐ Verbalization of appropriate action to take for pain control
- ☐ Demonstration of understanding of how weight control and exercise can influence cardiac disease

Key interventions

- Assess the patient's level of knowledge and readiness to learn about risk factor modification.

- Discuss the patient's risk factors and emphasize importance of modifying these behaviors.
- Instruct the patient to stop activity and rest when chest pain occurs.
- Teach the patient correct technique for self-administering prescribed sublingual nitrates.
- Discuss importance of stopping smoking.
- Refer the patient to appropriate support groups, such as smoking-cessation classes, and other self-help resources.
- Explain importance of weight management. Initiate dietary consultation for additional patient education.
- Explain role of stress in cardiac disease. Teach relaxation techniques.
- Discuss activity limitations and the need for regular exercise.
- Teach the patient about prescribed medications, including names, purposes, dosages, and common adverse effects.

Cardiac arrhythmias

Abnormalities of heart rate or rhythm caused by conduction system disturbances; they include abnormalities of impulse formation, impulse conduction, or both.

NURSING DIAGNOSIS

High risk for decreased cardiac output related to abnormal heart rhythm

DESIRED PATIENT OUTCOME

The patient will maintain an acceptable heart rate and rhythm

Outcome measurement criteria

- ☐ Heart rate of 60 to 100 beats/minute while the patient is at rest
- ☐ Acceptable heart rhythm
- ☐ Absence of dyspnea, syncope, and chest pain

Key interventions

- Monitor heart rate every 4 hours. Report irregularities.
- Evaluate heart rhythm every 4 hours through auscultation, telemetry, or both. Report irregularities.
- Monitor respiratory status for dyspnea.
- Instruct the patient to report dyspnea, dizziness, or chest pain immediately.
- Teach the patient correct technique for taking pulse.
- Instruct the patient to avoid straining during bowel movements. Offer stool softeners, if needed.

- Explain prescribed medication regimen, including antiarrhythmic therapy.
- Provide adequate rest between activities to prevent overexertion.

NURSING DIAGNOSIS

Anxiety related to perceived threat of death

DESIRED PATIENT OUTCOME

The patient will demonstrate abated signs of anxiety

Outcome measurement criteria

- ☐ Verbalization of concerns and fears
- ☐ Verbalization of realistic prognosis
- ☐ Relaxed facial expression and posture
- ☐ Demonstration of breathing techniques that promote relaxation during anxiety-provoking situations
- ☐ Demonstration of desire to reduce anxiety by learning about medical condition

Key interventions

- Assess the patient for signs and symptoms of anxiety, including verbal cues.
- Encourage the patient to verbalize concerns and fears.
- Teach breathing techniques that promote relaxation.
- Assist the patient in identifying and describing feelings and sources of anxiety.
- Encourage the patient to participate in diversional activities.
- Minimize anxiety-producing events.
- Encourage the patient to ask questions and learn about medical condition.

- Provide timely and accurate information. Answer questions honestly.

Cardiac surgery

Surgical intervention to correct a cardiac disorder, such as coronary artery occlusion, valvular disease, or congenital defect.

NURSING DIAGNOSIS

High risk for anxiety related to impending surgery and postoperative recovery

DESIRED PATIENT OUTCOME

The patient will express tolerance of anxiety related to cardiac surgery and postoperative recovery

Outcome measurement criteria

- ☐ Verbalization of concerns and fears
- ☐ Verbalization of understanding of surgical procedure and postoperative care
- ☐ Relaxed facial expression and posture
- ☐ Demonstration of relaxation techniques to help control anxiety
- ☐ Demonstration of correct techniques for coughing, deep breathing, and splinting the incision

Key interventions

- Assess the patient for signs and symptoms of anxiety, including verbal cues.
- Encourage the patient to express concerns and fears.
- Explain preoperative and postoperative care, including transfer to intensive care unit and subsequent return to medical-surgical unit.

- Teach correct techniques for coughing, deep breathing, and splinting.
- Teach relaxation techniques, such as deep breathing and guided imagery.
- Maintain environment conducive to relaxation.

NURSING DIAGNOSIS

Impaired physical mobility related to postoperative pain

DESIRED PATIENT OUTCOME

The patient will maintain functional mobility

Outcome measurement criteria

☐ Demonstration of increased mobility

☐ Verbalization of adequate pain control

☐ Participation in self-care activities

☐ Absence of complications of immobility, such as pneumonia, venous stasis, skin breakdown, and thrombus formation

Key interventions

- Provide adequate pain management.
- Assess the patient's functioning and mobility and document improvements daily.
- Administer pain medication, as prescribed, before the patient participates in activities.
- Observe for signs of complications, such as fever, increased lung consolidation, warmth and tenderness in legs, and skin breakdown.
- Teach the patient correct techniques for transferring in and out of bed.

- Explain importance of movement in preventing complications.
- Provide reassurance during movement.
- Encourage the family to assist the patient in changing position at least every 2 hours.

NURSING DIAGNOSIS

Ineffective breathing pattern related to incisional pain and decreased lung expansion

DESIRED PATIENT OUTCOME

The patient will demonstrate an acceptable breathing pattern

Outcome measurement criteria

- ☐ Respiratory rate and depth within normal ranges
- ☐ Verbalization of adequate pain control
- ☐ Absence of adventitious lung sounds
- ☐ Arterial blood gas (ABG) values within normal ranges
- ☐ Demonstration of correct incentive spirometry technique
- ☐ Demonstration of ability to cough, deep breathe, and splint the incision
- ☐ Verbalization of ability to breathe comfortably

Key interventions

- Assess respirations, lung sounds, and accessory muscle use at least every 4 hours.
- Teach the patient correct techniques for coughing, deep breathing, and splinting.
- Teach the patient correct use of incentive spirometry, and encourage its use every 2 hours.

- Encourage use of position that allows maximum lung expansion. For instance, lean the patient over padded overbed table, or keep patient in semi-Fowler's position.
- Provide adequate rest between breathing exercises to avoid fatigue.
- Monitor ABG results. Report significant changes to the physician.
- Provide supplemental oxygen, as prescribed and needed.
- Teach breathing techniques that promote relaxation, to decrease discomfort.

NURSING DIAGNOSIS

High risk for infection related to inflammation secondary to surgical trauma

DESIRED PATIENT OUTCOME

The patient will remain free of infection

Outcome measurement criteria

- ☐ Oral temperature at or below 99.0° F (37.2° C)
- ☐ White blood cell (WBC) count within normal range
- ☐ Absence of erythema, tenderness, and purulent drainage at incision site
- ☐ Approximation of wound edges
- ☐ Negative wound cultures

Key interventions

- Measure oral temperature at least every 4 hours.
- Monitor WBC count for increases that suggest infection. Report significant changes to the physician.
- Assess wound for signs of infection during each shift.

- Obtain wound cultures, as ordered, and monitor results.
- Consult the infection control practitioner, as needed.

NURSING DIAGNOSIS

High risk for ineffective management of therapeutic regimen related to required life-style modifications and perceived barriers to change

DESIRED PATIENT OUTCOME

The patient and family will demonstrate adequate skills for and knowledge of required follow-up care

Outcome measurement criteria

- ☐ Verbalization of activity limitations and the need to obtain adequate rest after discharge
- ☐ Verbalization of required dietary modifications
- ☐ Demonstration of correct wound management technique
- ☐ Verbalization of prescribed medication regimen
- ☐ Verbalization of signs and symptoms to report to physician

Key interventions

- Assess the patient's and family's knowledge regarding follow-up care and readiness to learn.
- Instruct the patient to increase activity gradually to avoid fatigue.
- Explain activity limitations, including avoidance of driving for 4 to 6 weeks and avoidance of heavy lifting.
- Explain that sexual activity may be contraindicated for up to 4 weeks. Check with the physician for specific recommendations.

- Initiate dietary consultation for patient education about dietary modifications.
- Instruct the patient to report the following signs and symptoms of infection to the physician: chest discomfort; fever; rapid pulse rate; or redness, pain, odorous wound drainage, or swelling at the incision site.
- Teach correct wound care technique. Stress handwashing as primary method to prevent infection.
- Provide information on cardiac support groups.
- Provide instruction about anticoagulant therapy, if the patient has had cardiac valve surgery.
- Discuss importance of notifying all medical and dental practitioners before undergoing any procedures, if the patient has had cardiac valve surgery.
- Encourage the family to participate in teaching sessions whenever possible.

Congestive heart failure

Complex clinical syndrome in which the heart cannot maintain adequate cardiac output.

NURSING DIAGNOSIS

Altered cardiopulmonary tissue perfusion related to inadequate cardiac output

DESIRED PATIENT OUTCOME

The patient will demonstrate improved cardiopulmonary tissue perfusion

Outcome measurement criteria

- ☐ Heart rate and blood pressure within normal ranges
- ☐ Warm and normally dry skin
- ☐ Decrease in dyspnea, fatigue, dizziness, and cool, clammy skin
- ☐ Decrease in jugular vein distention

Key interventions

- Assess apical rate and rhythm and blood pressure at least every 4 hours. Stay especially alert for new onset of S_3 (third heart sound), systolic murmur, or hypotension, which may indicate decreasing cardiac output. Report changes to the physician.
- Monitor the patient for jugular vein distention, dyspnea, and dizziness at least every 4 hours. Assess skin color and temperature.
- Maintain bed rest. Elevate head of bed 30 to 60 degrees to promote breathing.

- Provide adequate rest after self-care activities, diagnostic procedures, and visits.
- Monitor laboratory results for evidence of drug toxicity, particularly digitalis toxicity.

NURSING DIAGNOSIS

Impaired gas exchange related to altered oxygen supply

DESIRED PATIENT OUTCOME

The patient will demonstrate improved gas exchange

Outcome measurement criteria

- ☐ Respiratory rate of 12 to 20 breaths/minute
- ☐ Decrease in or absence of dyspnea, orthopnea, pallor, and cyanosis
- ☐ Demonstration of effective cough and expectoration of secretions
- ☐ Partial pressure of arterial oxygen (PaO_2) and carbon dioxide ($PaCO_2$) within normal ranges
- ☐ Clear lung sounds

Key interventions

- Monitor respiratory rate and depth and lung sounds at least every 4 hours.
- Observe for signs and symptoms of impaired ventilation, including restlessness, confusion, dyspnea, tachycardia, and cyanosis.
- Reposition the patient every 2 hours to promote mobilization of secretions.
- Lean the patient over padded overbed table to promote breathing, if necessary.
- Monitor arterial blood gas values, pulse oximetry values, and pulmonary function studies.

- Administer supplemental oxygen, as prescribed.
- Teach the patient correct techniques for coughing, deep breathing, and expectorating secretions.

NURSING DIAGNOSIS

Fluid volume excess related to ventricular failure and venous congestion secondary to congestive heart failure

DESIRED PATIENT OUTCOME

The patient will demonstrate resolution of fluid volume excess

Outcome measurement criteria

- ☐ Absence of peripheral and sacral edema
- ☐ Absence of jugular vein distention
- ☐ Absence of dyspnea, cough, orthopnea, and paroxysmal nocturnal dyspnea
- ☐ Clear lung sounds
- ☐ Return of weight to baseline
- ☐ Urine specific gravity between 1.005 and 1.010
- ☐ Verbalization of ability to breathe more easily

Key interventions

- Assess the patient for signs of dependent and sacral edema.
- Assess lung sounds at least every 4 hours. Stay alert for moist crackles (rales), indicating increasing pulmonary congestion.
- Weigh the patient at same time each day and document results.

- Observe the patient for signs of hypoxia, including dyspnea, cough, orthopnea, and paroxysmal nocturnal dyspnea.
- Observe the patient for jugular vein distention and signs of respiratory difficulty, which indicate fluid retention.
- Measure and record fluid intake and output during each shift.
- Evaluate and report fluid balance to the physician.
- Test urine specific gravity every 8 hours. Monitor serum electrolyte levels and report significant changes to the physician.
- Maintain fluid restrictions and sodium-restricted diet, as ordered.
- Explain importance of fluid and dietary restrictions to the patient to promote compliance. Encourage participation in monitoring fluid intake.
- Administer diuretics, as prescribed, and document the patient's response.

NURSING DIAGNOSIS

Activity intolerance related to fatigue and dyspnea

DESIRED PATIENT OUTCOME

The patient will tolerate a gradual increase in activity

Outcome measurement criteria

- ☐ Blood pressure, heart rate, and respiratory rate within acceptable limits during and after activity
- ☐ Verbalization of ability to tolerate activity
- ☐ Absence of severe dyspnea
- ☐ Demonstration of ability to perform activities of daily living to tolerance level

Key interventions

- Monitor vital signs before and after activity.
- Maintain bed rest or chair rest with feet elevated to decrease dependent edema.
- Provide regular position changes and range-of-motion exercises during bed rest.
- Provide bedside commode and shower chair to minimize fatigue.
- Encourage participation in self-care activities to tolerance level.
- Keep wheelchair nearby when patient ambulates, in case of fatigue, dyspnea, or chest pain.
- Allow adequate rest between activities.
- Provide positive reinforcement for increasing stamina.

NURSING DIAGNOSIS

Altered nutrition: less than body requirements related to decreased appetite and dietary restrictions

DESIRED PATIENT OUTCOME

The patient will maintain adequate nutritional intake

Outcome measurement criteria

- ☐ Demonstration of ability to maintain prescribed caloric intake
- ☐ Demonstration of improved appetite
- ☐ Participation in food selection, within dietary restrictions
- ☐ Serum albumin and protein levels within normal ranges

Key interventions

- Weigh the patient daily and document results.

- Monitor fluid intake and output and percentage of solid foods consumed at each meal.
- Monitor serum albumin and electrolyte levels. Report significant changes to the physician.
- Discuss dietary restrictions and food preferences with the patient.
- Explain importance of reducing dietary sodium and fat. Provide list of high-sodium foods to avoid, and suggest alternative seasonings, such as lemon juice and herbs.
- Position the patient comfortably during meals to promote easier breathing.
- Offer small, frequent feedings and high-calorie supplements, as indicated.
- Encourage family members to visit at mealtime to enhance meal enjoyment.
- Initiate dietary consultation for additional patient education.

NURSING DIAGNOSIS

Powerlessness related to effects of chronic illness on lifestyle

DESIRED PATIENT OUTCOME

The patient will verbalize a feeling of having regained control over the current health situation

Outcome measurement criteria

- ☐ Verbalization of concerns and fears about current health status
- ☐ Participation in decisions about care and treatment
- ☐ Participation in self-care activities to tolerance level
- ☐ Verbalization of feelings of having regained control over current health situation

- ☐ Verbalization of acceptance of required life-style changes
- ☐ Verbalization of specific strategies to reduce anxiety and manage chronic illness

Key interventions

- Encourage the patient to express feelings.
- Allow time for the patient to discuss concerns.
- Maintain nonjudgmental approach. Accept that feelings of powerlessness are normal in patients with chronic illness.
- Offer reassurance when the patient expresses feelings of powerlessness.
- Encourage participation in self-care activities.
- Allow the patient to participate in decisions about care and treatment whenever possible.
- Encourage the family to support the patient without being controlling.
- Ensure that the patient's spiritual needs are being met. Contact the chaplain or clergy of choice, if the patient desires.

Femoral-popliteal bypass

Surgical revascularization procedure in which a graft is placed to relieve signs and symptoms of acute or chronic ischemia in legs.

NURSING DIAGNOSIS

Fear related to impending surgery and postoperative recovery

DESIRED PATIENT OUTCOME

The patient will express less fear about the surgery and postoperative concerns

Outcome measurement criteria

- ☐ Verbalization of concerns and fears
- ☐ Verbalization of decreased fear
- ☐ Verbalization of understanding of surgical procedure and postoperative care
- ☐ Relaxed facial expression and posture
- ☐ Demonstration of relaxation techniques to help control fear
- ☐ Demonstration of correct techniques for coughing, deep breathing, and incentive spirometry

Key interventions

- Assess the patient for signs and symptoms of fear and anxiety, including verbal cues.
- Encourage the patient to express concerns and fears.

- Explain all preoperative and postoperative care routines, including transfer to intensive care unit and subsequent return to medical-surgical unit.
- Teach relaxation techniques, such as deep breathing and guided imagery.
- Maintain an environment conducive to relaxation.
- Teach correct techniques for coughing, deep breathing, and incentive spirometry. Observe return demonstration.

NURSING DIAGNOSIS

High risk for infection related to inflammation secondary to surgical trauma

DESIRED PATIENT OUTCOME

The patient will remain free of infection

Outcome measurement criteria

- ☐ Oral temperature at or below 99.0° F (37.2° C)
- ☐ White blood cell (WBC) count within normal range
- ☐ Absence of erythema, tenderness, and purulent drainage at incision site
- ☐ Approximation of wound edges
- ☐ Negative wound cultures

Key interventions

- Administer antibiotics, as prescribed, and document their effectiveness.
- Measure oral temperature at least every 4 hours.
- Monitor WBC count for increases that suggest infection. Report significant changes to the physician.
- Assess wound for signs of infection during each shift.

- Obtain wound cultures, as ordered, and monitor results.
- Instruct the patient to observe incision site for signs of infection for up to 90 days after discharge because prior tissue hypoxia increases risk of infection.
- Consult the infection control practitioner, as needed.

NURSING DIAGNOSIS

Pain related to inflammation secondary to surgical tissue trauma

DESIRED PATIENT OUTCOME

The patient will experience relief from pain

Outcome measurement criteria

☐ Verbalization of adequate pain relief

☐ Relaxed facial expression and muscle tone

☐ Vital signs within normal ranges

☐ Verbalization of ability to get adequate sleep

Key interventions

- Assess the patient for signs and symptoms of pain, including increased blood pressure, facial grimaces, splinting, shallow breathing, irritability, and restlessness.
- Explain management of postoperative pain, including meaning of *p.r.n.*
- Encourage the patient to request pain medication before pain becomes severe.
- Discuss use of around-the-clock pain medication schedule with the physician to achieve greater pain control.
- Teach the patient correct use of patient-controlled analgesia pump, if applicable.

- Use additional pain control methods, such as relaxation, music, and guided imagery, as an adjunct to pain medication.
- Monitor and document effectiveness of pain medication.
- Consult the physician and clinical pharmacist if pain management is ineffective.

NURSING DIAGNOSIS

High risk for peripheral neurovascular dysfunction related to reduced arterial blood flow secondary to ischemia of legs

DESIRED PATIENT OUTCOME

The patient will demonstrate adequate arterial blood flow of the legs

Outcome measurement criteria

☐ Presence of peripheral pulses in legs

☐ Absence of ischemic pain in legs

☐ Normal skin color and temperature in legs

☐ Absence of numbness and tingling in legs

Key interventions

- Assess peripheral pulses at least every 4 hours. (Use Doppler instrument if pulses cannot be palpated.) Document presence or absence of pulses and their intensity. Mark location of pulses with indelible marker to promote consistent comparisons.
- Assess legs for color, temperature, and capillary filling time every 4 hours. Observe skin for mottling or color changes, which suggest decreased perfusion.

- Assess surgical site for masses, ecchymosis, skin changes, and bleeding, which may indicate graft disruption.
- Monitor for signs and symptoms of hypotension, which could cause graft to collapse. Provide fluid replacement, as prescribed.
- Monitor hemoglobin and hematocrit values for evidence of blood loss.
- Avoid knee hyperextension and pressure on graft site.
- Use bed cradle to decrease pressure from linens.
- Instruct the patient to report ischemic pain, numbness, or tingling immediately.

NURSING DIAGNOSIS

Impaired physical mobility related to surgery and previous ischemic pain

DESIRED PATIENT OUTCOME

The patient will demonstrate increased physical mobility

Outcome measurement criteria

- ☐ Demonstration of increased physical mobility
- ☐ Verbalization of adequate pain control
- ☐ Demonstration of willingness to participate in self-care activities
- ☐ Verbalization of knowledge of positioning restrictions
- ☐ Absence of complications of immobility, including pneumonia, venous stasis, thrombus formation, and skin breakdown

Key interventions

- Provide adequate pain control. Provide pain medication, as prescribed, before activities.

- Elevate head of bed 30 to 60 degrees.
- Instruct the patient to avoid hyperextending knee, crossing legs, sitting longer than 20 minutes, and wearing clothing that may restrict blood flow.
- Encourage the patient to do range-of-motion exercises with unaffected extremities three to four times daily.
- Encourage participation in self-care activities.
- Explain importance of postoperative movement in preventing complications.
- Assist the patient with gradual increases in activity, such as transfer to chair, ambulation to bathroom, and ambulation in hallway.
- Offer positive reinforcement for efforts to increase mobility.

Hypertension

Intermittent or sustained elevation in blood pressure above 140/90 mm Hg.

NURSING DIAGNOSIS

Pain (headache) related to increased cerebrovascular pressure secondary to hypertension

DESIRED PATIENT OUTCOME

The patient will experience relief from pain

Outcome measurement criteria

☐ Verbalization of relief from pain

☐ Relaxed facial expression and muscle tone

☐ Vital signs within normal ranges

Key interventions

- Assess quality of pain. Evaluate for associated signs and symptoms, such as nausea, vomiting, and nosebleed.
- Investigate complaint of pain by assessing blood pressure and neurologic status to detect signs of intracranial hemorrhage.
- Administer analgesics, as prescribed.
- Encourage the patient to request pain medication before pain becomes severe.
- Provide ice packs, as desired, to relieve pain.
- Teach relaxation techniques, such as deep breathing and guided imagery.
- Maintain quiet environment with low lights and minimal stimulation.

- Instruct the patient to avoid sudden changes in position and jarring movements.
- Limit activities and visitors.
- Provide stool softeners to help prevent constipation.
- Instruct the patient to avoid Valsalva maneuver.

NURSING DIAGNOSIS

High risk for altered cerebral tissue perfusion related to impaired circulation

DESIRED PATIENT OUTCOME

The patient will demonstrate adequate cerebral tissue perfusion

Outcome measurement criteria

- ☐ Absence of alterations in level of consciousness (LOC) or orientation
- ☐ Blood pressure within acceptable range
- ☐ Vital signs within normal ranges
- ☐ Absence of headaches or dizziness

Key interventions

- Assess vital signs every 4 hours. Report significant changes to the physician.
- Assess neurologic status, including LOC, pupil reaction, and ability to move extremities.
- Administer antihypertensive medications, as prescribed, and document the patient's response.
- Instruct the patient to report headaches, dizziness, and vision changes immediately.
- Elevate head of bed 30 to 60 degrees.

- Monitor fluid therapy and fluid intake and output to evaluate fluid balance. Administer diuretics, as prescribed.
- Encourage progressive ambulation. Observe for orthostatic hypotension during ambulation.
- Instruct the patient to rest frequently to prevent fatigue.

NURSING DIAGNOSIS

Ineffective management of therapeutic regimen related to health beliefs

DESIRED PATIENT OUTCOME

The patient will follow a program for treating hypertension

Outcome measurement criteria

- ☐ Verbalization of personal beliefs about hypertension and its management
- ☐ Verbalization of intention to reduce hypertension risk factors
- ☐ Participation in developing plan to integrate hypertension treatment into daily life
- ☐ Demonstration of desire to use available resources
- ☐ Verbalization of understanding of hypertension
- ☐ Verbalization of behaviors that contribute to hypertension
- ☐ Demonstration of correct techniques for taking pulse and blood pressure
- ☐ Verbalization of role of regular exercise and weight management in controlling blood pressure

Key interventions

- Explain nature of hypertension and treatment plan.
- Encourage the patient to discuss personal beliefs about hypertension. Include the family in discussion, as appropriate.
- Discuss implications of ineffective hypertension management, emphasizing potential cardiovascular complications and cerebrovascular accident.
- Teach the patient about prescribed medications and importance of taking them even when feeling well.
- Discuss impotence as a possible adverse effect of antihypertensive medications (for male patient).
- Clarify misconceptions about hypertension and its treatment.
- Encourage the patient and family to ask questions.
- Include the family in teaching sessions as much as possible.
- Teach the patient to avoid taking over-the-counter medications unless the physician approves.
- Assist the patient and family in developing a manageable routine for integrating hypertension treatment into their life-styles. Consider cultural and financial factors as well as family dynamics.
- Encourage use of affirmations and positive thought processes as an additional hypertension management method.
- Assist the patient in making appropriate nutritional choices while hospitalized.
- Initiate dietary consultation for nutritional counseling. Reinforce the dietitian's instructions.
- Provide information on dietary guidelines after discharge. Include instructions about holiday meals, dining out, and nutritious fast-food options.

- Explain importance of stopping smoking and controlling weight, if applicable, to help prevent complications of hypertension.
- Instruct the patient to report headache, dizziness, vision changes, and faintness to the primary health care practitioner.
- Teach the patient and family correct techniques for taking pulse and blood pressure.
- Provide ample printed material for the patient to refer to at home.
- Provide information on appropriate community classes and support groups.

NURSING DIAGNOSIS

High risk for noncompliance with treatment plan related to the patient's value system

DESIRED PATIENT OUTCOME

The patient will demonstrate compliance with the treatment plan

Outcome measurement criteria

- ☐ Verbalization of factors that influence compliance
- ☐ Verbalization of intention to comply with treatment plan
- ☐ Demonstration of basic level of compliance

Key interventions

- Elicit the patient's reasons for noncompliance.
- Encourage the patient to express concerns and fears about hypertension and treatment plan.
- Maintain nonjudgmental approach. Avoid defensive behaviors.

- Assist the patient in identifying specific areas of non-compliance.
- Stress positive aspects of compliance, especially prevention of life-threatening complications of hypertension.
- Acknowledge the patient's right to choose not to comply with treatment plan.
- Provide positive reinforcement for compliant behavior.
- Encourage strong family support and use of support groups to promote ongoing compliance.

Pacemaker insertion

Surgical implantation of electronic device in subcutaneous pocket below clavicle, used to stimulate heart muscle to maintain or control heart rate. Catheter is placed in contact with heart using transvenous approach.

NURSING DIAGNOSIS

Fear related to impending surgery and postoperative recovery

DESIRED PATIENT OUTCOME

The patient will verbalize a decrease in fear regarding the surgery and postoperative concerns

Outcome measurement criteria

- ☐ Verbalization of concerns and fears
- ☐ Verbalization of decrease in fear
- ☐ Demonstration of understanding of surgical procedure and postoperative care
- ☐ Relaxed facial expression and posture
- ☐ Demonstration of relaxation techniques that help reduce fear

Key interventions

- Assess the patient for signs and symptoms of fear and anxiety, including verbal cues.
- Encourage the patient to express concerns and fears.
- Explain all preoperative and postoperative care routines, including transfer to intensive care unit and subsequent return to medical-surgical unit.

- Teach relaxation techniques, including deep breathing and guided imagery.
- Maintain environment conducive to relaxation.

NURSING DIAGNOSIS

High risk for decreased cardiac output related to possible pacemaker malfunction

DESIRED PATIENT OUTCOME

The patient will maintain an acceptable heart rate and rhythm

Outcome measurement criteria

- □ Heart rate above 60 beats/minute
- □ Blood pressure within normal range
- □ Acceptable heart rhythm
- □ Absence of dizziness, syncope, palpitations, fatigue, shortness of breath, and chest pain

Key interventions

- Assess the patient and pacemaker unit at least once every 4 hours. Observe for signs of decreased cardiac output, such as heart rate below 60 beats/minute, decreased blood pressure, dizziness, and cool, pale skin.
- Obtain 12-lead electrocardiogram (ECG), as ordered.
- Monitor ECG for evidence of adequate pacemaker sensing, capturing, and pacing, which indicate proper pacemaker function.
- Advise the patient to report chest pain, dizziness, or palpitations immediately.
- Elevate head of bed 30 to 45 degrees. Limit the patient's movement until fibrosis occurs at insertion site (to

prevent lead displacement), if passive lead placement was used.

- Provide limited range-of-motion exercise for other extremities until the patient begins progressive activity.

NURSING DIAGNOSIS

High risk for infection related to inflammation secondary to invasive procedure

DESIRED PATIENT OUTCOME

The patient will remain free of infection

Outcome measurement criteria

- ☐ Oral temperature at or below 99.0° F (37.2° C)
- ☐ White blood cell (WBC) count within normal range
- ☐ Absence of erythema, tenderness, and purulent drainage at incision site
- ☐ Approximation of wound edges
- ☐ Negative wound cultures

Key interventions

- Administer prophylactic antibiotics, as prescribed, and document their effectiveness.
- Measure oral temperature at least every 4 hours.
- Monitor WBC count for increases that may indicate infection. Report significant changes to the physician.
- Assess pacemaker site for signs of infection during each shift.
- Perform wound care, as ordered, using strict aseptic technique. Be aware that infection in pacemaker pocket may travel down wires to heart.

- Do not change primary dressing without a physician's order.
- Obtain wound cultures, as ordered, and monitor results.
- Consult the infection control practitioner, as needed.

NURSING DIAGNOSIS

Pain related to inflammation secondary to surgical tissue trauma

DESIRED PATIENT OUTCOME

The patient will experience relief from pain

Outcome measurement criteria

☐ Verbalization of adequate pain relief

☐ Relaxed facial expression and muscle tone

☐ Vital signs within normal ranges

Key interventions

- Assess the patient for signs and symptoms of pain, including increased blood pressure, facial grimaces, splinting, shallow breathing, irritability, and restlessness.
- Explain management of postoperative pain, including meaning of *p.r.n.*
- Encourage the patient to request pain medication before pain becomes severe.
- Use additional pain control methods, including relaxation, music, and guided imagery, as adjuncts to medication.
- Monitor and document effectiveness of pain medication.
- Consult the physician and clinical pharmacist if pain management is ineffective.

NURSING DIAGNOSIS

Altered health maintenance related to lack of knowledge regarding surgery and follow-up care

DESIRED PATIENT OUTCOME

The patient will verbalize knowledge of surgery and related follow-up care

Outcome measurement criteria

- ☐ Verbalization of purpose and function of pacemaker
- ☐ Verbalization of signs and symptoms to report
- ☐ Description of activity allowances and limitations
- ☐ Verbalization of awareness of electromagnetic hazards
- ☐ Demonstration of correct technique for pacemaker care
- ☐ Identification of importance of follow-up care

Key interventions

- Assess the patient's level of knowledge of and readiness to learn about follow-up care.
- Explain purpose and basic function of pacemaker. Describe type of pacemaker the patient has and established settings.
- Teach the patient to report signs and symptoms of pacemaker malfunction–dizziness, weakness, and pulse rate below pacemaker's set rate–to the primary health care practitioner.
- Instruct the patient to avoid traveling and driving for 4 weeks after pacemaker insertion. Explain that the patient may resume normal recreational activity, except contact sports.

- Discuss environmental hazards of electromagnetic power sources. Reassure the patient that most household appliances are safe, provided they are in proper working order.
- Teach the patient to recognize and report signs and symptoms of infection, including fever, chills, drainage, redness, swelling, and pain.
- Explain the need to protect pacemaker site by avoiding constricting clothing and direct physical contact at site.
- Instruct the patient to carry an identification card. Provide Medic-Alert application.
- Teach the patient and family correct technique for caring for pacemaker site. Observe return demonstration.

Percutaneous transluminal coronary angioplasty (PTCA)

Invasive, nonsurgical procedure in which balloon-tipped catheter is passed into partially blocked coronary artery; under fluoroscopic guidance, balloon is inflated to open arterial lumen and relieve obstruction.

NURSING DIAGNOSIS

Fear related to lack of knowledge of procedure and perceived threat of death

DESIRED PATIENT OUTCOME

The patient will demonstrate decreased fear

Outcome measurement criteria

- ☐ Verbalization of concerns and fears
- ☐ Verbalization of realistic prognosis
- ☐ Relaxed facial expression and posture
- ☐ Use of breathing techniques that promote relaxation during anxiety-provoking situations
- ☐ Demonstration of desire to learn about medical condition and treatment to help decrease fear

Key interventions

- Assess the patient for signs and symptoms of anxiety and fear, including verbal cues.
- Encourage the patient to verbalize concerns and fears.
- Assist the patient in identifying and describing feelings and sources of anxiety and fear.

- Minimize anxiety-producing events.
- Describe procedure and sensations the patient may feel during it, including pressure during catheter insertion and flushing or nausea during dye injection. Explain that procedure usually lasts 2 to 5 hours.
- Explain postprocedural care, including bed rest for 6 to 8 hours, sandbag or pressure dressing application to puncture site, and frequent vital sign and peripheral pulse assessment.
- Teach breathing techniques that promote relaxation.
- Encourage the patient to ask questions and learn about medical condition and PTCA.
- Provide timely and accurate information. Answer questions honestly.

NURSING DIAGNOSIS

High risk for altered peripheral tissue perfusion related to possible thrombus formation secondary to PTCA

DESIRED PATIENT OUTCOME

The patient will maintain adequate peripheral tissue perfusion

Outcome measurement criteria

☐ Presence of pulses distal to cannulation site

☐ Warm and normally dry skin

☐ Coagulation studies within normal ranges

Key interventions

- Assess and document presence and intensity of peripheral pulses.

- Assess skin color and temperature. Observe for cyanosis, cool and clammy skin, and decreased capillary filling time, which indicate decreased perfusion.
- Assess for signs and symptoms of hematoma in affected extremity, including ecchymosis, swelling, redness, and pain. Instruct the patient to report these signs and symptoms immediately.
- Teach the patient to keep affected extremity extended and immobile for 6 to 8 hours after procedure. Maintain bed rest during this time.
- Maintain pressure dressing or sandbag over puncture site, as ordered, to prevent bleeding.
- Monitor coagulation studies and report abnormalities to the physician.

NURSING DIAGNOSIS

High risk for injury related to abnormal heart rhythm secondary to PTCA

DESIRED PATIENT OUTCOME

The patient will remain free of injury from complications of PTCA

Outcome measurement criteria

- ☐ Vital signs within normal ranges
- ☐ Blood pressure within normal range
- ☐ Acceptable heart rhythm
- ☐ Absence of dyspnea, chest pain, or syncope

Key interventions

- Monitor heart rate every 4 hours. Report abnormalities to the physician.

- Auscultate heart sounds for diminished or extra sounds. Report irregularities.
- Monitor respiratory status for diminished breath sounds, adventitious lung sounds, and dyspnea. Report abnormalities.
- Instruct the patient to report chest pain, dyspnea, or dizziness immediately.
- Monitor peripheral pulses for presence or absence and intensity.
- Assess skin color and temperature.
- Maintain fluid therapy, as prescribed.
- Monitor fluid intake and output. Report urine output below 30 ml/hour.

NURSING DIAGNOSIS

Ineffective management of therapeutic regimen related to lack of information regarding follow-up care

DESIRED PATIENT OUTCOME

The patient will verbalize knowledge of postprocedural care

Outcome measurement criteria

- ☐ Verbalization of importance of follow-up care
- ☐ Verbalization of activity limitations
- ☐ Verbalization of risk factors requiring modification
- ☐ Description of names, purposes, dosage, and common adverse effects of prescribed medications
- ☐ Verbalization of signs and symptoms to report

Key interventions

- Assess the patient's knowledge about follow-up care and readiness to learn.
- Discuss concerns or fears raised by the patient or family.
- Teach the patient about activity limitations. Explain that most patients can return to work within 1 week after discharge.
- Discuss risk factors for cardiac disease, including excessive weight, smoking, stress, and sedentary lifestyle.
- Assist the patient in identifying risk factors that require modification.
- Teach the patient about importance of avoiding nicotine, which increases risk of restenosis after PTCA.
- Instruct the patient to report chest pain, dizziness, or dyspnea immediately.
- Review names, purposes, dosages, and common adverse effects of prescribed medications.
- Teach the patient about importance of follow-up care. Explain the need for periodic treadmill testing.
- Provide pamphlets and instruction sheets the patient can refer to after discharge.

Peripheral vascular disease

Chronic arterial insufficiency characterized by inadequate arterial blood flow, leading to hypoperfusion and ischemia.

NURSING DIAGNOSIS

Altered peripheral tissue perfusion related to reduced arterial blood flow

DESIRED PATIENT OUTCOME

The patient will demonstrate improved peripheral tissue perfusion

Outcome measurement criteria

- ☐ Maintenance of or improvement in peripheral pulses
- ☐ Adequate skin color and temperature
- ☐ Adequate capillary filling time
- ☐ Absence of numbness and tingling
- ☐ Demonstration of ability to move affected extremity

Key interventions

- Assess peripheral pulses at least every 4 hours, and document their presence or absence and intensity. (Use Doppler instrument if unable to palpate pulses.) Mark location of pulses with indelible marker to promote consistent comparisons.
- Assess skin color and temperature and capillary filling time every 4 hours. Observe for mottling or color changes that indicate decreased perfusion.
- Elevate head of bed 30 degrees.
- Use bed cradle to decrease pressure from linens.

- Instruct the patient to report ischemic pain, numbness, or tingling immediately.
- Avoid direct application of heat to affected extremities.
- Instruct the patient to perform leg exercises twice daily to promote circulation.
- Encourage ambulation to level of tolerance.
- Monitor coagulation studies and report abnormalities to the physician.

NURSING DIAGNOSIS

Pain related to decreased circulation to extremities

DESIRED PATIENT OUTCOME

The patient will verbalize adequate control of pain

Outcome measurement criteria

- ☐ Verbalization of tolerable level of pain
- ☐ Relaxed facial expression and muscle tone
- ☐ Vital signs within normal ranges

Key interventions

- Assess type and severity of pain. Document pain level, using 1-to-10 scale.
- Advise the patient to request pain medication before pain becomes severe.
- Monitor and document effectiveness of pain medication.
- Position the patient for maximum comfort. Do not raise knee gatch, elevate extremity, or permit hip flexion because these actions interfere with arterial flow.
- Provide passive and active range-of-motion exercise, unless contraindicated.

NURSING DIAGNOSIS

High risk for impaired skin integrity related to decreased circulation in affected extremities

DESIRED PATIENT OUTCOME

The patient will maintain intact skin over affected extremities

Outcome measurement criteria

- ☐ Skin of normal dryness and color
- ☐ Adequate skin turgor
- ☐ Absence of signs of impaired skin integrity
- ☐ Demonstration of appropriate skin care

Key interventions

- Inspect skin for redness, blisters, decreased turgor, edema, and excessive dryness during each shift.
- Keep skin clean and dry.
- Lubricate excessively dry skin with oil or lotion.
- Change the patient's position every 2 hours.
- Assist the patient in maintaining adequate hydration.
- Monitor hemoglobin, hematocrit, serum protein, and serum albumin values for evidence of dehydration and poor nutritional status.
- Advise the patient to control itching by pressing on area or applying ice.
- Teach the patient and family to inspect the patient's skin frequently.

NURSING DIAGNOSIS

Activity intolerance related to ischemic pain

DESIRED PATIENT OUTCOME

The patient will tolerate activity at gradually increasing levels

Outcome measurement criteria

- □ Verbalization of desire to increase activity
- □ Participation in self-care activities
- □ Demonstration of ability to increase ambulation without pain
- □ Blood pressure and heart rate within normal ranges during activity

Key interventions

- Discuss activity limitations with the patient and family.
- Administer pain medication, as prescribed, before activity.
- Encourage participation in activities to tolerance level. Instruct the patient to rest if intermittent claudication occurs.
- Explain importance of planned rest periods in preventing fatigue and maintaining balance between oxygen supply and demand.
- Monitor the patient's response to increasing activity.
- Encourage the patient to develop plan for balancing activity with rest after discharge.

Thrombophlebitis

Acute vascular condition characterized by thrombus formation and inflammation in deep or superficial vein.

NURSING DIAGNOSIS

Pain related to inflammation

DESIRED PATIENT OUTCOME

The patient will experience relief from pain

Outcome measurement criteria

- ☐ Verbalization of relief from pain
- ☐ Relaxed facial expression and muscle tone
- ☐ Vital signs within normal ranges

Key interventions

- Assess and document location and quality of pain.
- Administer pain medication, as prescribed, and document the patient's response.
- Encourage the patient to request pain medication before pain becomes severe.
- Measure and document girth of affected extremity daily.
- Elevate affected extremity above level of right atrium. Do not use knee gatch because this may impede circulation.
- Apply warm, moist compresses, as ordered. Do not leave compresses in place longer than 20 minutes.
- Apply antiembolism stockings, as ordered. Remove stockings for 1 hour each shift and then reapply.

- Consult the physician and clinical pharmacist if pain control is ineffective.

NURSING DIAGNOSIS

Altered peripheral tissue perfusion related to interruption in venous blood flow

DESIRED PATIENT OUTCOME

The patient will demonstrate adequate peripheral tissue perfusion

Outcome measurement criteria

- ☐ Maintenance of or improvement in peripheral pulses
- ☐ Adequate skin temperature and color
- ☐ Absence of pain

Key interventions

- Assess for presence and intensity of peripheral pulses in affected extremity at least every 4 hours.
- Assess for changes in skin color and temperature. Notify the physician of significant changes.
- Measure girth of affected extremity daily. Mark spot where measurements are taken to promote consistent measurements.
- Administer anticoagulant therapy, as prescribed. Monitor for signs of bleeding, bruising, and other adverse effects.
- Assist the patient in gradual initiation of activity.
- Instruct the patient to avoid nicotine to help prevent further vascular constriction.
- Instruct the patient to avoid crossing legs, wearing constrictive clothing, or standing for prolonged periods.

NURSING DIAGNOSIS

High risk for impaired skin integrity related to venous stasis

DESIRED PATIENT OUTCOME

The patient will maintain intact skin

Outcome measurement criteria

- ☐ Skin of normal dryness and color
- ☐ Adequate skin turgor
- ☐ Absence of signs of impaired skin integrity
- ☐ Demonstration of appropriate skin care

Key interventions

- Inspect skin for redness, blisters, decreased turgor, edema, and abnormal dryness during each shift.
- Change the patient's position every 2 hours.
- Keep the patient's skin clean and dry.
- Lubricate excessively dry skin with oil or lotion.
- Assist the patient in maintaining adequate hydration.
- Monitor hemoglobin, hematocrit, serum protein, and serum albumin values for signs of dehydration and poor nutritional status.
- Advise the patient to control itching by pressing on area or applying ice.
- Teach the patient and family to inspect the patient's skin frequently.

NURSING DIAGNOSIS

High risk for impaired gas exchange related to possible embolism

DESIRED PATIENT OUTCOME

The patient will remain free of pulmonary embolism

Outcome measurement criteria

- ☐ Absence of dyspnea, chest pain, and tachypnea
- ☐ Clear lung sounds
- ☐ Partial pressure of arterial oxygen (PaO_2) and carbon dioxide ($PaCO_2$) within normal ranges

Key interventions

- Assess the patient for signs and symptoms of pulmonary embolism, including acute dyspnea, tachypnea, chest pain, extreme anxiety, pallor, and hemoptysis. Notify the physician of these findings immediately.
- Administer anticoagulant therapy, as prescribed.
- Monitor arterial blood gas values and report abnormalities.
- Auscultate lung sounds at least every 4 hours.
- Encourage the patient to turn, cough, and deep breathe every 2 hours.
- Offer calm reassurance to decrease anxiety.
- Maintain bed rest during acute episodes.

NURSING DIAGNOSIS

Health-seeking behaviors related to prevention of recurrent thrombus formation

DESIRED PATIENT OUTCOME

The patient will verbalize knowledge of preventive measures and follow-up care

Outcome measurement criteria

- ☐ Verbalization of disease process
- ☐ Verbalization of preventive measures
- ☐ Demonstration of correct application of antiembolism stockings
- ☐ Demonstration of appropriate skin care
- ☐ Verbalization of anticoagulant therapy precautions

Key interventions

- Assess the patient's knowledge about medical condition and preventive measures as well as readiness to learn.
- Explain importance of follow-up care.
- Teach correct technique for applying antiembolism stockings. Observe return demonstration.
- Encourage the patient to avoid constricting clothing, such as garters, girdles, and knee-high stockings with elastic bands.
- Explain importance of stopping smoking, if applicable.
- Discourage oral contraceptive use.
- Instruct the patient to avoid temperature extremes and massaging affected extremity.
- Teach appropriate skin care. Observe return demonstration.
- Review names, purposes, dosages, and common adverse effects of prescribed medications.
- Discuss anticoagulant therapy precautions. Instruct the patient to avoid taking aspirin and over-the-counter medications unless the physician approves.
- Explain importance of follow-up visits and laboratory studies to evaluate effectiveness of therapy.

- Instruct the patient to notify the primary health care practitioner of unusual bleeding, including bleeding from gums or nose, increased menstrual flow, and hematuria.
- Instruct the patient to use soft-bristled toothbrush and avoid water-jet tooth cleaners.
- Initiate dietary consultation for nutritional counseling.
- Provide the patient with Medic-Alert application.

Adult respiratory distress syndrome (ARDS)

Acute syndrome characterized by pulmonary edema and acute respiratory failure resulting from increased alveolocapillary membrane permeability; lungs become noncompliant, wet, heavy, congested, hemorrhagic, and unable to diffuse oxygen.

NURSING DIAGNOSIS

Impaired gas exchange related to disruption of alveolocapillary membrane secondary to ARDS

DESIRED PATIENT OUTCOME

The patient will regain adequate gas exchange

Outcome measurement criteria

- ☐ Arterial blood gas (ABG) and pulse oximetry values within acceptable range for the patient's condition
- ☐ Partial pressure of arterial oxygen (PaO_2) of 50 to 60 mm Hg
- ☐ Arterial oxygen saturation (SaO_2) above 90%
- ☐ Clear lung sounds
- ☐ Vital capacity and tidal volume optimal for the patient's condition

Key interventions

- Administer oxygen therapy, as prescribed.

- Assess breath sounds every 4 hours, or more often if the patient's condition warrants.
- Monitor vital signs every 4 hours. Observe for tachypnea and tachycardia.
- Monitor ABG and pulse oximetry values. Notify the physician if PaO_2 or partial pressure of carbon dioxide ($PaCO_2$) changes by more than 15 mm Hg or if SaO_2 falls below 90%.
- Assess neurologic status, including level of consciousness and orientation. Report subtle changes to the physician.
- Monitor cardiac status every 4 hours for signs of arrhythmias. Report suspected arrhythmias to the physician.
- Review pulmonary function studies to detect changes in vital capacity and tidal volume.
- Position the patient for maximum comfort and lung expansion.
- Change the patient's position every 2 hours to help mobilize secretions.

NURSING DIAGNOSIS

High risk for ineffective breathing pattern related to hypoxia and fatigue secondary to ARDS

DESIRED PATIENT OUTCOME

The patient will regain an effective breathing pattern

Outcome measurement criteria

☐ Respiratory rate of 12 to 20 breaths/minute

☐ Unobstructed breathing

☐ Decreased use or nonuse of accessory breathing muscles

☐ ABG and pulse oximetry values within normal ranges

☐ Absence of dyspnea, cyanosis, and tachycardia

☐ Absence of need for mechanical ventilatory support

☐ Verbalization of ability to breathe comfortably

Key interventions

- Administer bronchodilators and expectorants, as prescribed.
- Assess and document respiratory rate and depth every 4 hours.
- Auscultate breath sounds every 4 hours for signs of increasing pulmonary congestion.
- Monitor ABG and pulse oximetry values. Report significant changes to the physician.
- Observe for accessory muscle use, nasal flaring, dyspnea, cyanosis, and tachypnea.
- Observe for restlessness, confusion, and irritability.
- Teach the patient how to perform pursed-lip breathing to maximize lung expansion.
- Maintain the patient in semi-Fowler's position.
- Assist with self-care activities to conserve the patient's energy.
- Schedule rest periods between activities.
- Encourage the family to respect the patient's need for rest.

NURSING DIAGNOSIS

High risk for aspiration related to increased secretions and airway impairment

DESIRED PATIENT OUTCOME

The patient will show no signs of aspiration of secretions, food, or other substances, and will show no signs of infection or other sequelae of aspiration

Outcome measurement criteria

☐ Patent airway

☐ Mobilization and expectoration of secretions

☐ Absence of signs of aspiration

☐ Oral temperature at or below 99.0° F (37.2° C)

☐ White blood cell (WBC) count within normal range

Key interventions

- Monitor respiratory status closely.
- Assess for gag and swallow reflexes.
- Observe type, amount, and character of secretions. Note the patient's ability to expectorate secretions.
- Monitor temperature at least every 4 hours.
- Monitor WBC count.
- Elevate head of bed at least 30 degrees during meals; maintain elevation for at least 1 hour after meals.
- Teach correct techniques for coughing, deep breathing, and expectorating secretions. Observe return demonstration.
- Provide humidification if secretions are thick. Suction when necessary to maintain clear airway.

NURSING DIAGNOSIS

Anxiety related to air hunger secondary to ARDS

DESIRED PATIENT OUTCOME

The patient will demonstrate abated signs of anxiety

Outcome measurement criteria

- ☐ Respiratory rate and depth within normal ranges
- ☐ Vital signs within normal ranges
- ☐ Verbalization of decreasing anxiety
- ☐ Relaxed facial expression and muscle tone
- ☐ Demonstration of breathing techniques that promote relaxation

Key interventions

- Assess for signs and symptoms of anxiety.
- Encourage the patient to verbalize concerns and fears.
- Implement measures to reduce dyspnea, such as semi-Fowler's positioning, leaning the patient on padded overbed table, administering supplemental oxygen, as ordered, and providing rest periods.
- Minimize anxiety-producing events.
- Teach breathing techniques that promote relaxation.
- Encourage the patient to ask questions and learn about ARDS.
- Provide timely and accurate information. Answer questions honestly.

NURSING DIAGNOSIS

Ineffective individual coping related to sudden onset of life-threatening condition

DESIRED PATIENT OUTCOME

The patient will demonstrate positive coping techniques

Outcome measurement criteria

- ☐ Verbalization of feelings
- ☐ Demonstration of expected emotional responses
- ☐ Communication of needs to staff
- ☐ Verbalization of techniques that reduce anxiety
- ☐ Demonstration of adequate problem-solving and decision-making skills
- ☐ Demonstration of appropriate use of support systems

Key interventions

- Discuss coping strategies the patient has used during difficult situations in past. Encourage the patient to use positive strategies to deal with current illness.
- Assist the patient in identifying needs clearly.
- Assist the patient in identifying methods that reduce anxiety, such as relaxation techniques and music therapy.
- Allow the patient to participate in decisions about care.
- Use open communication to promote expression of feelings.
- Maintain nonjudgmental approach toward the patient and family.
- Encourage the family to support the patient during times of stress.
- Ensure that spiritual needs of the patient and family are being met. Contact the chaplain or clergy of choice if the patient or family desires.

Asthma

Airway disorder characterized by recurrent episodes of paroxysmal dyspnea, with wheezing caused by bronchospasm; results from hyperactivity of tracheobronchial smooth muscle, leading to airway inflammation, mucosal swelling, increased secretions, and air trapping.

NURSING DIAGNOSIS

Ineffective airway clearance related to bronchospasm

DESIRED PATIENT OUTCOME

The patient will maintain a patent airway

Outcome measurement criteria

- ☐ Patent airway
- ☐ Clear lung sounds
- ☐ Absence of dyspnea and cyanosis
- ☐ Demonstration of ability to breathe without obstruction

Key interventions

- Administer corticosteroids and bronchodilators, as prescribed, and document the patient's response.
- Assess lung sounds and respiratory rate and effort at least every 4 hours. Document presence of rhonchi, crackles, and wheezes.
- Observe for dyspnea, tachypnea, accessory muscle use, cyanosis, and dry or productive cough.
- Assess skin turgor and mucous membranes for signs of dehydration.

- Elevate head of bed 45 to 90 degrees, if tolerated.
- Encourage fluid intake of up to 2,500 ml/24 hours, unless contraindicated.
- Monitor fluid intake and output during each shift.
- Withhold dairy products, which increase mucus viscosity.
- Help the patient lean on padded overbed table, if indicated.
- Change the patient's position every 2 hours to mobilize secretions.
- Teach correct techniques for coughing, deep breathing, and expectorating secretions. Observe return demonstration.

NURSING DIAGNOSIS

Ineffective breathing pattern related to anxiety and lung hyperinflation

DESIRED PATIENT OUTCOME

The patient will regain an effective breathing pattern

Outcome measurement criteria

- ☐ Respiratory rate of 12 to 20 breaths/minute
- ☐ Decreased use or nonuse of accessory breathing muscles
- ☐ Arterial blood gas (ABG) and pulse oximetry values within normal ranges
- ☐ Verbalization of ability to breathe comfortably
- ☐ Absence of dyspnea, shortness of breath, cyanosis, tachycardia, and substernal tightness

Key interventions

- Administer bronchodilators and expectorants, as prescribed.
- Assess and document respiratory rate and depth every 4 hours.
- Observe for accessory muscle use, nasal flaring, dyspnea, shortness of breath, cyanosis, and tachypnea.
- Auscultate breath sounds every 4 hours for wheezing, crackles, and rhonchi.
- Monitor ABG and pulse oximetry values. Report significant changes to the physician.
- Keep the patient in semi-Fowler's position.
- Instruct the patient to report difficulty breathing immediately.
- Teach pursed-lip breathing to improve bellows action of lungs.
- Encourage participation in self-care activities to tolerance level.
- Use nasal cannula to deliver oxygen during meals, if oxygen usually is delivered by mask.
- Schedule rest periods between activities.
- Encourage the family to respect the patient's need for rest.

NURSING DIAGNOSIS

Anxiety related to difficulty breathing

DESIRED PATIENT OUTCOME

The patient will demonstrate abated signs of anxiety

Outcome measurement criteria

☐ Normal respiratory rate and depth

☐ Verbalization of decrease in anxiety

☐ Relaxed facial expression and muscle tone

☐ Demonstration of breathing techniques that promote relaxation

Key interventions

- Assess for signs and symptoms of anxiety.
- Encourage the patient to verbalize concerns and fears.
- Minimize anxiety-producing events.
- Stay with the patient during episodes of bronchospasm or intense coughing. Offer reassurance to help reduce anxiety.
- Teach breathing techniques that promote relaxation.
- Position the patient to promote optimal respiration.
- Encourage the patient to ask questions and learn about medical condition.
- Provide timely and accurate information. Answer questions honestly.

NURSING DIAGNOSIS

High risk for infection related to steroid therapy

DESIRED PATIENT OUTCOME

The patient will demonstrate a decreased risk for infection and for spreading infection to others

Outcome measurement criteria

☐ Oral temperature at or below 99.0° F (37.2° C)

☐ White blood cell (WBC) count within normal range

- ☐ Verbalization of signs and symptoms of infection
- ☐ Demonstration of correct techniques for coughing, deep breathing, and expectorating and disposing of secretions

Key interventions

- Measure temperature every 4 hours.
- Observe for diaphoresis, chills, and change in mucus color or consistency.
- Monitor WBC count and report changes to the physician.
- Encourage fluid intake of up to 2,500 ml/24 hours, unless contraindicated, to maintain hydration and liquefy secretions.
- Reposition the patient every 2 hours to help mobilize secretions.
- Teach correct techniques for coughing, deep breathing, and expectorating and disposing of secretions. Observe return demonstration.
- Instruct the patient to cover mouth when coughing or sneezing.
- Caution the patient to avoid contact with people who have respiratory tract infections.
- Instruct the patient to report fever, congestion, changes in sputum color and consistency, chills, aches, and diaphoresis to the primary health care practitioner.
- Administer prophylactic antibiotics, as prescribed, and document the patient's response.

NURSING DIAGNOSIS

Altered health maintenance related to lack of knowledge regarding preventive measures and follow-up care for asthma

DESIRED PATIENT OUTCOME

The patient and family will verbalize knowledge of preventive measures and follow-up care for asthma

Outcome measurement criteria

- ☐ Verbalization of understanding of disease process
- ☐ Verbalization of factors that may precipitate asthma
- ☐ Verbalization of names, purposes, dosages, and common adverse effects of prescribed medications
- ☐ Demonstration of correct breathing techniques
- ☐ Demonstration of proper use and care of breathing equipment

Key interventions

- Assess the patient's knowledge and readiness to learn about medical condition and required follow-up care
- Describe disease process and precipitating factors.
- Assist the patient in identifying factors that may worsen or precipitate asthma, including emotional stress, fatigue, dust, pet dander, allergens, and pollen.
- Review names, purposes, dosages, and common adverse effects of antibiotics, bronchodilators, corticosteroids, or other prescribed medications.
- Teach correct technique for using inhaler. Observe return demonstration.
- Provide instruction about breathing equipment and its use. Observe return demonstration.
- Teach pursed-lip breathing and breathing techniques that promote relaxation.
- Explain importance of adequate hydration, nutrition, and planned rest periods in recovery.
- Instruct the patient to stop smoking, if applicable, and to avoid people who are smoking.

- Discuss importance of exercising to tolerance level.
- Instruct the patient to prevent spread of infection through good handwashing, correct disposal of secretions, and avoidance of exposure to infected people.
- Refer the patient and family to appropriate support groups and community classes to attend after discharge.
- Provide application for Medic-Alert identification.

Chronic airway limitation

Collective term for group of diseases, such as chronic bronchitis and emphysema, characterized by recurrent airflow obstruction usually involving expiratory phase of respiration.

NURSING DIAGNOSIS

Ineffective airway clearance related to increased secretions and bronchospasm

DESIRED PATIENT OUTCOME

The patient will maintain a patent airway

Outcome measurement criteria

- ☐ Patent airway
- ☐ Decreased secretions
- ☐ Clear lung sounds
- ☐ Absence of dyspnea and cyanosis

Key interventions

- Administer bronchodilators and antibiotics, as prescribed, and document the patient's response.
- Assess lung sounds and respiratory rate and effort at least every 4 hours. Document presence of rhonchi, crackles, and wheezes.
- Observe for dyspnea, tachypnea, fever, cyanosis, and cough.
- Assess skin turgor and mucous membranes for signs of dehydration.
- Elevate head of bed 45 to 90 degrees, if tolerated.

- Encourage fluid intake of up to 2,500 ml/24 hours, unless contraindicated.
- Monitor fluid intake and output during each shift.
- Withhold dairy products, which increase mucus viscosity.
- Help the patient lean on padded overbed table, if indicated.
- Change the patient's position every 2 hours to help mobilize secretions.
- Teach correct techniques for coughing, deep breathing, and expectorating secretions. Observe return demonstration.

NURSING DIAGNOSIS

Impaired gas exchange related to airway obstruction

DESIRED PATIENT OUTCOME

The patient will regain adequate gas exchange

Outcome measurement criteria

- ☐ Arterial blood gas (ABG) values within normal ranges for the patient's condition
- ☐ Partial pressure of arterial oxygen (PaO_2) of 50 to 60 mm Hg
- ☐ Arterial oxygen saturation (SaO_2) above 90%
- ☐ Return of vital capacity and tidal volume to baseline values
- ☐ Clear lung sounds

Key interventions

- Administer oxygen, as prescribed.

- Assess breath sounds at least every 4 hours, or more often if condition warrants.
- Assess neurologic status, including level of consciousness and orientation. Report subtle changes to the physician.
- Monitor vital signs every 4 hours. Observe for tachypnea and tachycardia.
- Monitor ABG and pulse oximetry values. Notify the physician if PaO_2 or partial pressure of carbon dioxide ($PaCO_2$) changes by more than 15 mm Hg or if SaO_2 falls below 90%.
- Monitor cardiac status every 4 hours for signs of arrhythmias. Report arrhythmias to the physician.
- Review pulmonary function studies for changes in vital capacity and tidal volume.
- Position the patient for maximum comfort and lung expansion.
- Change the patient's position every 2 hours to help mobilize secretions.

NURSING DIAGNOSIS

Ineffective breathing pattern related to anxiety and lung hyperinflation

DESIRED PATIENT OUTCOME

The patient will regain an effective breathing pattern

Outcome measurement criteria

☐ Respiratory rate of 12 to 20 breaths/minute

☐ Unobstructed breathing

☐ Decreased use of accessory breathing muscles

☐ ABG values within normal ranges

- □ Verbalization of ability to breathe more comfortably
- □ Absence of dyspnea, shortness of breath, cyanosis, tachycardia, and substernal tightness
- □ Clear chest X-ray

Key interventions

- Administer bronchodilators and expectorants, as prescribed.
- Assess and document respiratory rate and depth every 4 hours.
- Observe for accessory muscle use, nasal flaring, dyspnea, shortness of breath, cyanosis, and tachypnea.
- Auscultate breath sounds every 4 hours for crackles, wheezes, and rhonchi.
- Monitor ABG and pulse oximetry values. Report significant changes to the physician.
- Instruct the patient to report difficulty breathing immediately.
- Keep the patient in semi-Fowler's position.
- Teach pursed-lip breathing to improve bellows action of lungs.
- Encourage participation in self-care activities to tolerance level.
- Schedule rest periods between activities.
- Encourage the family to respect the patient's need for rest.

NURSING DIAGNOSIS

Altered nutrition: less than body requirements related to shortness of breath and decreased appetite

DESIRED PATIENT OUTCOME

The patient will increase nutritional intake to an adequate level

Outcome measurement criteria

- ☐ Maintenance of weight, or weight increase to within normal range
- ☐ Maintenance of adequate caloric intake
- ☐ Participation in food selection
- ☐ Serum albumin and protein levels within normal ranges
- ☐ Absence of shortness of breath during meals

Key interventions

- Obtain baseline weight on admission and then weigh the patient daily to determine progress.
- Monitor serum protein and albumin levels to help assess nutritional status.
- Position the patient for optimal lung expansion.
- Consult the dietitian for appropriate calorie count and nutritional assessment, if necessary.
- Discuss food preferences. Encourage the patient to participate in food selection.
- Plan rest periods before meals.
- Perform respiratory hygiene and mouth care before meals, to clear airway.
- Offer small, frequent feedings of nutritious foods and fluids.
- Use nasal cannula to deliver oxygen during meals, if oxygen usually is delivered by mask.
- Provide high-protein, low-carbohydrate supplements.
- Instruct the patient to avoid gas-forming foods, which worsen abdominal distention and shortness of breath.

- Encourage the family to bring favorite foods from home, within dietary restrictions.
- Encourage the family to visit during meals to enhance meal enjoyment.

NURSING DIAGNOSIS

Sleep pattern disturbance related to stimulant effects of medication, anxiety, and shortness of breath

DESIRED PATIENT OUTCOME

The patient will regain the ability to obtain adequate sleep

Outcome measurement criteria

- ☐ Verbalization of factors that influence ability to sleep
- ☐ Demonstration of ability to fall asleep easily
- ☐ Verbalization of ability to get adequate sleep
- ☐ Decrease in shortness of breath

Key interventions

- Assess the patient's normal sleep pattern.
- Explain factors that may influence ability to sleep.
- Encourage the patient to verbalize concerns and fears.
- Implement measures to minimize shortness of breath, such as positioning and oxygen therapy.
- Organize care activities to allow uninterrupted sleep.
- Instruct the patient to perform deep-breathing and coughing exercises before going to sleep to decrease nocturnal dyspnea.
- Monitor the patient's ability to sleep at night, noting length of uninterrupted sleep, respiratory rate and depth, and breath sounds.

- Collaborate with the physician, if necessary, to change dosages or administration schedule of prescribed bronchodilators to enhance rest.
- Teach the patient about relaxation techniques that promote sleep, such as deep breathing, guided imagery, and listening to soft music or nature sounds.

NURSING DIAGNOSIS

Powerlessness related to effects of chronic illness on life-style

DESIRED PATIENT OUTCOME

The patient will verbalize a feeling of having regained control over chronic illness

Outcome measurement criteria

- ☐ Verbalization of concerns and fears about health status
- ☐ Demonstration of ability to make decisions regarding care and treatment
- ☐ Participation in self-care activities to tolerance level
- ☐ Verbalization of feelings of having regained control over chronic illness
- ☐ Verbalization of acceptance of required life-style changes
- ☐ Verbalization of specific strategies for reducing anxiety and managing chronic illness

Key interventions

- Encourage the patient to express feelings about health status.
- Provide time to discuss concerns.

- Use nonjudgmental approach and avoid defensive behaviors. Accept that feelings of powerlessness are normal in patients with chronic illness.
- Offer reassurance during periods when the patient feels powerless.
- Encourage participation in self-care activities to tolerance level.
- Allow the patient to participate in decisions about care and treatment whenever possible.
- Encourage the family to support the patient without being controlling.
- Ensure that the patient's spiritual needs are being met. Contact the chaplain or clergy of choice if the patient desires.

Lung cancer

Neoplastic disease characterized by uncontrolled growth of anaplastic cells in lung.

NURSING DIAGNOSIS

Pain related to inflammation secondary to destruction of normal cells

DESIRED PATIENT OUTCOME

The patient will verbalize relief from pain

Outcome measurement criteria

- ☐ Verbalization of adequate relief from pain
- ☐ Relaxed facial expression and muscle tone
- ☐ Demonstration of ability to self-administer pain medication, if applicable

Key interventions

- Assess for signs and symptoms of pain, including increased blood pressure, facial grimaces, splinting, shallow respirations, restlessness, and irritability.
- Discuss pain control with the patient, family, and physician to develop effective pain management plan.
- Encourage the patient to request pain medication before pain becomes severe.
- Encourage use of patient-controlled analgesia (PCA) pump, if appropriate, to provide increased sense of control over pain. Teach the patient and family about PCA and correct use of equipment. Observe return demonstration. If the patient becomes unable to use PCA because of alterations in level of consciousness, ask

the physician to consider continuous analgesic infusion for maximum comfort.

- Use additional methods, such as relaxation, guided imagery, and music therapy, to help manage pain.
- Monitor and document effectiveness of pain management. Consult the physician and clinical pharmacist if pain management is ineffective.

NURSING DIAGNOSIS

Altered protection related to immunosuppression secondary to chemotherapy

DESIRED PATIENT OUTCOME

The patient will remain free of infection

Outcome measurement criteria

- ☐ Oral temperature at or below 99.0° F (37.2° C)
- ☐ White blood cell (WBC) count within normal range
- ☐ Negative blood cultures
- ☐ Adherence to isolation techniques

Key interventions

- Measure oral temperature at least every 8 hours.
- Monitor WBC for increases that suggest infection.
- Monitor blood cultures, as indicated.
- Implement reverse isolation, if indicated and ordered.
- Discuss reverse isolation guidelines with the patient and family to promote compliance.
- Practice diligent handwashing to prevent cross-contamination.
- Maintain strict aseptic technique when performing invasive procedures.

- Consult the infection control practitioner, if needed.

NURSING DIAGNOSIS

Ineffective breathing pattern related to discomfort and decreased lung expansion

DESIRED PATIENT OUTCOME

The patient will regain an effective breathing pattern

Outcome measurement criteria

- ☐ Respiratory rate of 12 to 20 breaths/minute
- ☐ Unobstructed breathing
- ☐ Decreased use or nonuse of accessory breathing muscles
- ☐ Arterial blood gas (ABG) values within normal ranges
- ☐ Arterial oxygen saturation (SaO_2) above 90%
- ☐ Verbalization of ability to breathe comfortably
- ☐ Absence of dyspnea, shortness of breath, cyanosis, tachycardia, and substernal tightness

Key interventions

- Assess and document respiratory rate and depth every 4 hours.
- Observe for accessory muscle use, nasal flaring, dyspnea, shortness of breath, cyanosis, and tachypnea.
- Auscultate breath sounds every 4 hours for wheezes, crackles, and rhonchi.
- Monitor ABG and pulse oximetry values.
- Maintain the patient in semi-Fowler's position.
- Instruct the patient to report difficulty breathing immediately.
- Teach pursed-lip breathing to maximize lung expansion.

- Encourage participation in self-care activities to tolerance level.
- Schedule rest periods between activities.
- Encourage the family to respect the patient's need for rest.

NURSING DIAGNOSIS

Ineffective airway clearance related to bronchial obstruction secondary to tumor

DESIRED PATIENT OUTCOME

The patient will maintain a patent airway

Outcome measurement criteria

- ☐ Patent airway
- ☐ Decrease in secretions
- ☐ Clear lung sounds
- ☐ Absence of dyspnea and cyanosis

Key interventions

- Assess lung sounds and respiratory rate and effort at least every 4 hours. Document presence of rhonchi, crackles, and wheezes.
- Observe for dyspnea, tachypnea, nasal stuffiness, fever, cyanosis, and cough.
- Assess skin turgor and mucous membranes for signs of dehydration.
- Elevate head of bed 45 to 90 degrees, if tolerated.
- Change the patient's position every 2 hours to help mobilize secretions.
- Teach correct techniques for coughing, deep breathing, and expectorating secretions. Observe return demonstration.

- Encourage fluid intake of up to 2,500 ml/24 hours, unless contraindicated.
- Monitor fluid intake and output during each shift.
- Withhold dairy products, which increase mucus viscosity.

NURSING DIAGNOSIS

Altered nutrition: less than body requirements, related to nausea, vomiting, and anorexia secondary to chemotherapy

DESIRED PATIENT OUTCOME

The patient will increase nutritional intake to an adequate level

Outcome measurement criteria

- ☐ Maintenance of weight, or weight increase
- ☐ Maintenance of adequate caloric intake
- ☐ Participation in food selection
- ☐ Serum albumin and protein levels within normal ranges
- ☐ Absence of severe nausea and vomiting
- ☐ Absence of lesions in oral mucous membrane (stomatitis)
- ☐ Verbalization of measures that help control nausea and vomiting
- ☐ Verbalization of importance of reporting significant weight loss to the primary health care practitioner

Key interventions

- Obtain baseline weight on admission and then weigh the patient every 2 weeks to determine progress.
- Assess bowel sounds during each shift.

- Monitor serum protein and albumin levels to help assess nutritional status.
- Administer antiemetics before chemotherapy, as prescribed.
- Position the patient for optimal lung expansion.
- Assess oral cavity and mucous membranes for stomatitis.
- Schedule rest periods before meals.
- Perform oral hygiene before meals, using mild mouthwash and viscous lidocaine.
- Consult the dietitian regarding appropriate calorie count and nutritional assessment, if necessary.
- Discuss food preferences. Encourage the patient to participate in food selection.
- Offer small, frequent feedings of nutritious soft foods and fluids.
- Use nasal cannula to deliver oxygen during meals, if oxygen usually is administered by mask.
- Encourage the family to bring favorite foods from home, within dietary restrictions.
- Encourage the family to visit during meals to enhance meal enjoyment.

NURSING DIAGNOSIS

Spiritual distress related to challenged beliefs secondary to terminal illness

DESIRED PATIENT OUTCOME

The patient will express a sense of increased spiritual comfort

Outcome measurement criteria

☐ Verbalization of source of spiritual distress

- ☐ Verbalization of feelings regarding current spiritual and religious beliefs
- ☐ Description of stages of grief
- ☐ Identification of current stage in grief
- ☐ Demonstration of effective strategies to ease spiritual distress
- ☐ Verbalization and seeking out of appropriate support systems, including family, friends, clergy, and cancer support groups

Key interventions

- Listen for verbal cues indicating spiritual distress, such as questioning meaning of life and death, expressing anger with God, and bargaining.
- Use active listening and acknowledge the patient's feelings and spiritual concerns.
- Encourage the patient to discuss specific religious beliefs, to gain further insight.
- Discuss grief process and associated stages. Help the patient identify current stage of grief.
- Encourage the patient to continue religious or spiritual practices during hospitalization to ease distress.
- Arrange for visits with the hospital chaplain or clergy of choice. Provide privacy during visits.

NURSING DIAGNOSIS

Caregiver role strain related to unpredictable course of illness

DESIRED PATIENT OUTCOME

The caregiver will develop positive strategies to deal with role strain

Outcome measurement criteria

- ☐ Identification of current stressors
- ☐ Verbalization of effect of role strain on daily life
- ☐ Verbalization of feelings regarding competing roles
- ☐ Demonstration of positive coping strategies to deal with role strain
- ☐ Verbalization of need for respite help and recreation
- ☐ Demonstration of acceptance of help from family, friends, or outside agencies to manage responsibilities

Key interventions

- Encourage the caregiver to discuss feelings and concerns.
- Discuss current stressors with the caregiver.
- Help the caregiver acknowledge and identify specific stressors that increase role strain.
- Use open, nonjudgmental approach to promote trusting relationship.
- Discuss coping skills the caregiver has used successfully in the past. Assist in adapting these skills to current situation.
- Discuss diversional activities and hobbies the caregiver enjoys. Explore ways to incorporate these into daily life.
- Identify areas of knowledge deficit. Provide information to increase knowledge and, thus, reduce strain.
- Assist the caregiver in identifying support systems, including family members, friends, religious institutions, and clergy.
- Consult social services department for information on community resources, such as Meals on Wheels, respite care, and hospice care.

Mechanical ventilation

Ventilation achieved through extrinsic means, used for patients whose breathing problems interfere with gas exchange and may result in apnea or respiratory failure; commonly begins during the patient's stay in intensive care unit (ICU) and continues after transfer to medical-surgical unit.

NURSING DIAGNOSIS

Ineffective airway clearance related to intubation and copious secretions

DESIRED PATIENT OUTCOME

The patient will maintain a patent airway

Outcome measurement criteria

☐ Patent airway

☐ Decrease in secretions

☐ Clear lung sounds

☐ Absence of dyspnea and cyanosis

Key interventions

- Assess lung sounds at least every 4 hours. Document presence of rhonchi, crackles, and wheezes.
- Observe for evidence that the patient is "fighting" ventilator, such as dyspnea, tachypnea, cyanosis, and restlessness.
- Observe quantity, color, odor, and consistency of secretions.
- Suction airway, as needed. Instill sterile saline solution into endotracheal tube or tracheostomy to liquefy secretions during suctioning.

- Reposition the patient at least every 2 hours to help mobilize secretions.
- Provide humidification to help keep secretions liquefied.

NURSING DIAGNOSIS

Ineffective breathing pattern related to neuromuscular involvement, inflammation, and decreased expansion of lungs

DESIRED PATIENT OUTCOME

The patient will regain an effective breathing pattern

Outcome measurement criteria

- ☐ Unobstructed breathing
- ☐ Decreased use of accessory breathing muscles
- ☐ Arterial blood gas (ABG) and pulse oximetry values within normal ranges
- ☐ Absence of dyspnea, cyanosis, and tachycardia
- ☐ Absence of signs of "fighting" the ventilator

Key interventions

- Assess and document respiratory rate and depth every 4 hours. Check ventilator settings frequently.
- Monitor ABG and pulse oximetry values. Report significant changes to the physician.
- Observe for accessory muscle use, nasal flaring, dyspnea, cyanosis, and tachycardia.
- Assess for signs of "fighting" the ventilator, which may indicate discrepancy between the patient's respiratory cycles and those of ventilator.

- Investigate possible reasons why patient is "fighting" the ventilator, such as pain, secretions, and fear. Intervene to treat cause, as appropriate.
- Check each ventilator connection for snug fit.
- Always leave ventilator alarms on.
- Implement prescribed measures to minimize risk of self-extubation, such as restraints and sedation.
- Reassure the patient to help decrease anxiety.

NURSING DIAGNOSIS

High risk for infection related to stasis of secretions and loss of respiratory defenses secondary to mechanical ventilation

DESIRED PATIENT OUTCOME

The patient will remain free of infection

Outcome measurement criteria

☐ Oral temperature at or below 99.0° F (37.2° C)

☐ White blood cell (WBC) count within normal range

☐ Absence of changes in sputum quality and odor

☐ Negative sputum cultures

☐ Absence of diaphoresis and chills

Key interventions

- Measure and document oral temperature every 4 hours.
- Assess for diaphoresis, chills, and changes in sputum quality and odor.
- Obtain sputum cultures and monitor results.
- Administer prophylactic antibiotics, as prescribed.
- Change all ventilator components that come into contact with the patient every 24 hours.

- Empty water from tubing periodically.

NURSING DIAGNOSIS

Fear related to dependence on mechanical ventilator

DESIRED PATIENT OUTCOME

The patient will demonstrate less fear of dependence on mechanical ventilator

Outcome measurement criteria

☐ Absence of restlessness and agitation

☐ Verbalization of decrease in fear

☐ Respiratory rate and depth within normal ranges

☐ Relaxed muscle tone

☐ Absence of signs of "fighting" the ventilator

☐ Absence of self-extubation

Key interventions

- Monitor the patient for signs of fighting the ventilator, such as increasing restlessness and agitation.
- Monitor respiratory rate, depth, and muscle tone for signs of increasing fear.
- Explain mechanical ventilation to the patient and family, using simple terms.
- Provide the patient with alternative communication method.
- Reassure the patient that ventilator alarms are always turned on to alert the staff to problems.
- Inform the patient that personnel are always available to meet the patient's needs.

- Teach the patient how to use the call and emergency lights. Keep these lights within the patient's reach at all times.
- Place the patient near nurses' station, if possible.
- Make frequent rounds to check on the patient, to help increase comfort and reduce fear, especially just after the patient's transfer from ICU.
- Encourage the patient and family to communicate their concerns to the staff.

NURSING DIAGNOSIS

Impaired verbal communication related to intubation

DESIRED PATIENT OUTCOME

The patient will maintain an effective level of communication

Outcome measurement criteria

- ☐ Demonstration of ability to use alternative method of communication
- ☐ Consistent communication of needs to staff
- ☐ Demonstration of satisfaction with chosen communication method

Key interventions

- Discuss communication impairment with the patient and family.
- Reassure the patient that acceptable communication method will be established immediately.
- Provide choice of communication methods, such as paper and pen, Magic Slate, picture board, poster with common questions, and use of gestures.

- Teach the patient how to use chosen communication method. Include the family in teaching sessions.
- Observe for signs of increasing frustration, withdrawal, or depression. Intervene promptly to correct problem.
- Reorient the patient as necessary.
- Speak to the patient in short, simple sentences, and allow time for response.
- Provide positive reinforcement to promote continued attempts at communication.

Pneumonia

Acute inflammation of respiratory bronchioles and alveolar spaces caused by infection.

NURSING DIAGNOSIS

Impaired gas exchange related to lung consolidation and increased secretions

DESIRED PATIENT OUTCOME

The patient will demonstrate adequate or improved gas exchange

Outcome measurement criteria

- ☐ Absent or diminished signs of hypoxia, such as restlessness, confusion, and irritability
- ☐ Absence of cyanosis
- ☐ Partial pressure of arterial oxygen (PaO_2) above 60 mm Hg
- ☐ Arterial blood gas (ABG) and pulse oximetry values within normal ranges for the patient's condition
- ☐ Heart rate within normal range
- ☐ Progressive improvement of chest X-rays

Key interventions

- Assess respiratory rate, depth, and pattern.
- Assess for changes in orientation and increasing restlessness.
- Monitor ABG values closely and report abnormalities to the physician.

- Assess skin color for cyanosis, particularly around lips and nail beds.
- Administer oxygen therapy, as prescribed.

NURSING DIAGNOSIS

Ineffective airway clearance related to increased secretions

DESIRED PATIENT OUTCOME

The patient will maintain a patent airway

Outcome measurement criteria

☐ Demonstration of ability to expectorate secretions

☐ Unobstructed breathing

☐ Clear breath sounds

☐ Consumption of adequate fluids

Key interventions

- Assess ability to mobilize secretions. If mobilization is inadequate, assist with positioning, suctioning, and chest percussion.
- Assess quality of breath sounds at least every 4 hours.
- Teach proper techniques for deep breathing, coughing, and incentive spirometry use. Encourage the patient to perform these techniques every hour while awake.
- Explain importance of increasing fluid intake to help liquefy secretions. Encourage fluid intake of at least 2,000 ml/24 hours, unless contraindicated. Encourage the family to offer plenty of fluids.

NURSING DIAGNOSIS

High risk for altered body temperature related to inflammation and invading organism

DESIRED PATIENT OUTCOME

The patient will maintain a body temperature within the normal range

Outcome measurement criteria

- ☐ Oral temperature at or below 99.0° F (37.2°C) for at least 48 hours
- ☐ White blood cell (WBC) count within normal range
- ☐ Negative sputum culture
- ☐ Decrease in sputum production

Key interventions

- Administer antibiotics, as prescribed, to achieve and maintain therapeutic blood drug levels.
- Measure oral temperature at least every 4 hours and whenever the patient has chills or diaphoresis.
- Monitor sputum cultures and WBC count to evaluate antibiotic effectiveness.
- Provide comfort measures, such as keeping the patient clean and dry and offering fluids.
- Administer antipyretics, as prescribed, and document the patient's response.

NURSING DIAGNOSIS

Pain related to pleural irritation and coughing

DESIRED PATIENT OUTCOME

The patient will experience relief from pain

Outcome measurement criteria

- ☐ Verbalization of relief from pain
- ☐ Relaxed facial expression and muscle tone
- ☐ Demonstration of correct splinting technique
- ☐ Demonstration of effective cough

Key interventions

- Assess for objective and subjective signs of discomfort.
- Teach the patient how to splint while coughing and deep breathing to minimize discomfort.
- Use appropriate positioning and relaxation techniques to reduce discomfort.
- Encourage the patient to verbalize discomfort so comfort measures can begin promptly.
- Pace activities to provide adequate rest.
- Administer analgesics, as prescribed, and evaluate and document effectiveness.

NURSING DIAGNOSIS

Ineffective management of therapeutic regimen related to lack of information about preventive measures and follow-up care

DESIRED PATIENT OUTCOME

The patient and family will verbalize knowledge of preventive measures and follow-up care

Outcome measurement criteria

- ☐ Demonstration of correct pulmonary hygiene techniques
- ☐ Verbalization of realistic plan of activity and rest

- ☐ Verbalization of signs and symptoms to report to the physician
- ☐ Verbalization of importance of adequate nutrition and fluid intake
- ☐ Verbalization of measures that help prevent disease recurrence
- ☐ Verbalization of names, purposes, dosages, and common adverse effects of discharge medications

Key interventions

- Teach deep-breathing and coughing techniques and correct tissue disposal. Observe return demonstration.
- Explain importance of adhering to prescribed medication regimen.
- Discuss importance of adequate food and fluid intake and adequate rest in promoting recovery.
- Discuss signs and symptoms to report to the physician, including elevated temperature, diaphoresis, difficulty breathing, persistent cough, and cold or influenza symptoms.
- Instruct the patient to avoid contact with people with respiratory tract infections.
- Teach the patient and family about importance of maintaining pulmonary hygiene after discharge.
- Advise the patient to receive influenza vaccines, unless contraindicated.

Thoracic surgery

Surgery involving chest-wall incision, such as thoracotomy, pneumonectomy, and lobectomy.

NURSING DIAGNOSIS

Fear related to impending surgery and postoperative recovery

DESIRED PATIENT OUTCOME

The patient will express decreased fear regarding surgery and postoperative recovery

Outcome measurement criteria

- ☐ Verbalization of concerns and fears
- ☐ Verbalization of basic understanding of surgery and postoperative care
- ☐ Relaxed facial expression and body posture
- ☐ Demonstration of relaxation techniques to help control fear
- ☐ Demonstration of correct techniques for deep breathing, coughing, and splinting incision

Key interventions

- Assess for signs and symptoms of fear and anxiety, including verbal cues.
- Encourage the patient to express concerns and fears.
- Explain preoperative and postoperative care.
- Teach correct coughing, deep-breathing, and splinting techniques. Observe return demonstration.

- Provide instruction about relaxation techniques, such as breathing exercises, guided imagery, and music therapy.
- Maintain calm environment.

NURSING DIAGNOSIS

Pain related to inflammation secondary to surgical tissue trauma

DESIRED PATIENT OUTCOME

The patient will experience relief from pain

Outcome measurement criteria

- ☐ Verbalization of relief from pain
- ☐ Relaxed facial expression and muscle tone
- ☐ Vital signs within normal ranges

Key interventions

- Assess for signs and symptoms of pain, including increased blood pressure, facial grimaces, shallow breathing, splinting, irritability, and restlessness.
- Explain management of postoperative pain, including meaning of *p.r.n.*
- Advise the patient to request pain medication before pain becomes severe.
- Use additional pain control methods, such as relaxation, music, and guided imagery.
- Monitor and document effectiveness of pain medication.
- Consult the physician and clinical pharmacist if pain management is ineffective.

NURSING DIAGNOSIS

Ineffective breathing pattern related to pain, fatigue, and chest tubes

DESIRED PATIENT OUTCOME

The patient will regain an effective breathing pattern

Outcome measurement criteria

- ☐ Respiratory rate of 12 to 20 breaths/minute
- ☐ Unobstructed breathing
- ☐ Verbalization of ability to breathe comfortably
- ☐ Decreased use of accessory breathing muscles
- ☐ Arterial blood gas (ABG) and pulse oximetry values within normal ranges
- ☐ Absence of dyspnea, shortness of breath, cyanosis, and tachycardia
- ☐ Intact chest drainage system, if applicable

Key interventions

- Administer pain medications, as prescribed.
- Assess and document respiratory rate and depth every 4 hours after initial postoperative period.
- Observe for accessory muscle use, nasal flaring, dyspnea, shortness of breath, cyanosis, and tachypnea.
- Auscultate breath sounds every 4 hours for wheezes, crackles, and rhonchi.
- Monitor chest tube system for proper suction or gravity, water seal, and air leaks.
- Monitor ABG and pulse oximetry values. Report significant changes to the physician.
- Assess for gastrointestinal distention, which could reduce lung expansion.

- Keep the patient in semi-Fowler's position.
- Instruct the patient to report difficulty breathing immediately.
- Teach pursed-lip breathing to maximize lung expansion.
- Encourage participation in self-care activities to tolerance level.
- Schedule rest periods between activities.
- Encourage the family to respect the patient's need for rest.

NURSING DIAGNOSIS

High risk for infection related to surgical tissue trauma

DESIRED PATIENT OUTCOME

The patient will remain free of infection

Outcome measurement criteria

☐ Oral temperature at or below 99.0° F (37.2° C)

☐ White blood cell (WBC) count within normal range

☐ Absence of erythema, tenderness, and purulent drainage at incision site

☐ Approximation of wound edges

☐ Negative wound cultures

Key interventions

- Measure oral temperature at least every 4 hours.
- Monitor WBC for increases that suggest infection. Report significant findings to the physician.
- Wash hands before and after contact with wound to help prevent spread of infection.

- Assess wound during each shift for signs of infection, including warmth, redness, tenderness, purulent drainage, and odor.
- Obtain wound cultures, as ordered, and monitor results.
- Consult the infection control practitioner, as needed.

NURSING DIAGNOSIS

Impaired physical mobility related to pain, fatigue, and chest tubes

DESIRED PATIENT OUTCOME

The patient will demonstrate improved physical mobility

Outcome measurement criteria

- ☐ Verbalization of tolerable pain level
- ☐ Demonstration of improved physical mobility
- ☐ Participation in self-care activities
- ☐ Absence of signs of complications of immobility, such as pneumonia, venous stasis, thrombus formation, and skin breakdown

Key interventions

- Discuss complications of postoperative immobility.
- Assess for signs and symptoms of pain, which could impair mobility.
- Administer pain medication before activity, as prescribed.
- Instruct the patient to report increasing pain to ensure prompt intervention.
- Teach the patient to perform active range-of-motion (ROM) exercises several times daily. If the patient cannot do these exercises, assist with passive ROM.

- Teach the patient how to splint incision when coughing or getting out of bed.
- Encourage the patient to ambulate. Assist during ambulation, as needed.
- Provide rest between activities to help prevent fatigue.
- Administer supplemental oxygen, as prescribed and needed.
- Maintain chest drainage system below level of insertion to prevent backflow.
- Reassure the patient that chest tube will not become dislodged.
- Monitor participation in self-care activities. Assist as necessary to conserve the patient's energy.

Tuberculosis

Chronic infectious disease affecting alveolar structure of lung, caused by various species of Mycobacterium.

NURSING DIAGNOSIS

High risk for infection transmission related to lack of knowledge and poor health practices

DESIRED PATIENT OUTCOME

The patient will verbalize understanding of the importance of refraining from practices that may lead to tuberculosis transmission

Outcome measurement criteria

- □ Verbalization of disease transmission modes
- □ Verbalization of practices that decrease disease transmission
- □ Demonstration of correct technique for coughing and disposing of secretions
- □ Demonstration of correct isolation technique to use when moving beyond hospital room

Key interventions

- Assess the patient's current knowledge about disease transmission.
- Assess for signs and symptoms of active tuberculosis infection, including sputum production, cough, increased temperature, chills, and night sweats.
- Explain disease transmission modes.
- Teach the patient to cough and sneeze into disposable tissues and to discard tissues in isolation trash bags.

- Observe pulmonary hygiene practices to verify understanding.
- Explain need for isolation and instruct the patient in proper use of tuberculosis mask.
- Emphasize importance of good handwashing in decreasing spread of infection.

NURSING DIAGNOSIS

Ineffective breathing pattern related to destruction of lung tissue

DESIRED PATIENT OUTCOME

The patient will regain an adequate breathing pattern

Outcome measurement criteria

- ☐ Respiratory rate of 12 to 20 breaths/minute
- ☐ Unobstructed breathing
- ☐ Decreased use of accessory breathing muscles
- ☐ Arterial blood gas (ABG) values within normal ranges
- ☐ Absence of dyspnea, cyanosis, and tachycardia

Key interventions

- Assess respiratory rate and depth every 4 hours.
- Monitor ABG values and report changes to the physician.
- Auscultate lung sounds every 4 hours for crackles, rhonchi, and wheezes.
- Observe for accessory muscle use, dyspnea, cyanosis, and tachypnea.
- Observe for restlessness, confusion, and irritability, which may indicate hypoxia.
- Elevate head of bed 45 degrees.

- Assist with activities of daily living to help conserve the patient's energy.
- Schedule rest periods between activities.

NURSING DIAGNOSIS

Altered nutrition: less than body requirements, related to fatigue and decreased appetite

DESIRED PATIENT OUTCOME

The patient will increase nutritional intake

Outcome measurement criteria

☐ Maintenance of or increase in weight

☐ Maintenance of adequate caloric intake

☐ Participation in food selection

☐ Serum albumin and protein levels within normal ranges

Key interventions

- Obtain baseline weight on admission and then weigh the patient daily to determine progress.
- Monitor serum protein and albumin levels to help assess nutritional status.
- Position the patient for optimal lung expansion.
- Discuss food preferences. Encourage the patient to participate in food selection.
- Consult the dietitian regarding appropriate calorie count and nutritional assessment, if necessary.
- Provide rest before meals.
- Perform respiratory hygiene and mouth care before meals to clear airway.
- Offer small, frequent feedings of high-carbohydrate, high-protein foods.

- Use nasal cannula to deliver oxygen therapy during meals.
- Monitor percentage of food the patient consumes at each meal.
- Encourage the family to bring favorite foods from home, within dietary restrictions.
- Encourage the family to visit during meals to enhance meal enjoyment.

NURSING DIAGNOSIS

High risk for noncompliance related to complexity of treatment

DESIRED PATIENT OUTCOME

The patient will verbalize the intention to comply with the treatment plan

Outcome measurement criteria

- ☐ Verbalization of factors that influence compliance
- ☐ Verbalization of importance of complying with treatment plan
- ☐ Verbalization of desire to adhere to treatment plan
- ☐ Demonstration of basic compliance
- ☐ Demonstration of correct technique for sputum disposal and placement of tuberculosis face mask
- ☐ Verbalization of importance of good hygiene and nutrition
- ☐ Verbalization of importance of follow-up medical appointments, chest X-rays, and blood tests

Key interventions

- Determine the patient's reasons for noncompliance.

- Assist in identifying specific areas of noncompliance.
- Encourage the patient to verbalize concerns and fears related to illness and treatment plan.
- Maintain nonjudgmental approach. Avoid defensive behaviors.
- Stress positive aspects of compliance, especially in preventing complications with chronic effects and stopping spread of tuberculosis to others.
- Provide positive reinforcement for compliant behavior.
- Consult social services department for assistance in identifying medical assistance and community services
- Arrange for follow-up care by a visiting nurse to promote compliance after discharge.
- Report required information to health department.
- Discuss names, purposes, dosages, and common adverse effects of prescribed medications. Stress importance of finishing all medications as prescribed. Teach the patient which adverse effects to report to the physician.
- Make appointment for the patient's next clinic or physician appointment before discharge.
- Emphasize importance of monthly sputum cultures until cultures are negative and then every 3 months for duration of therapy (possibly up to 24 months).

Appendicitis

Inflammation of vermiform appendix, usually acute; may be simple or perforated and typically necessitates surgery to remove appendix.

NURSING DIAGNOSIS

Anxiety related to pain, impending surgery, and lack of knowledge regarding postoperative care

DESIRED PATIENT OUTCOME

The patient will exhibit decreased anxiety

Outcome measurement criteria

- ☐ Verbalization of fears
- ☐ Verbalization of understanding of surgical procedure and postoperative care
- ☐ Relaxed facial expression and body posture
- ☐ Use of relaxation techniques to control anxiety
- ☐ Demonstration of correct techniques for coughing, deep breathing, and splinting

Key interventions

- Assess the patient for signs and symptoms of anxiety, including verbal cues.
- Encourage the patient to express fears.
- Explain all preoperative and postoperative care.
- Teach relaxation techniques, such as deep breathing and guided imagery.

- Maintain environment that is conducive to relaxation.
- Provide instruction in coughing, deep breathing, and splinting. Observe return demonstrations.
- Teach the patient or family member correct wound care technique. Observe return demonstration.
- Explain that activities, including walking and driving, will be increased gradually.
- Instruct the patient to report signs and symptoms of wound infection immediately.
- Emphasize importance of following discharge instructions.

NURSING DIAGNOSIS

Pain related to inflammation

DESIRED PATIENT OUTCOME

The patient will experience relief from pain

Outcome measurement criteria

☐ Verbalization of adequate pain relief

☐ Vital signs within normal ranges

☐ Relaxed facial expression and muscle tone

☐ Verbalization of ability to get adequate sleep

Key interventions

- Assess for signs and symptoms of pain, including increased blood pressure, facial grimaces, shallow breathing, and restlessness.
- Explain principles of pain management, including meaning of *p.r.n.*
- Monitor and document effectiveness of pain medication.

- Encourage the patient to request pain medication before pain becomes severe.
- Use additional pain control methods, such as relaxation, music, and guided imagery, as adjuncts to medication.

NURSING DIAGNOSIS

High risk for infection related to inflammation secondary to tissue trauma and risk of perforation

DESIRED PATIENT OUTCOME

The patient will remain free of infection

Outcome measurement criteria

- ☐ Oral temperature at or below 99.0° F (37.2° C)
- ☐ White blood cell (WBC) count within normal range
- ☐ Absence of erythema, purulent drainage, and tenderness at incision site
- ☐ Approximation of wound edges
- ☐ Soft, nontender abdomen

Key interventions

- Measure oral temperature at least every 4 hours.
- Assess abdomen for rigidity and tenderness, which suggest peritonitis.
- Monitor WBC count for increases that suggest infection, and report these to the physician.
- Assess wound for warmth, redness, drainage, tenderness, and odor during each shift.
- Obtain wound cultures, as needed, and monitor results.
- Consult the infection control practitioner, as needed.

Cholecystectomy

Surgical removal of gallbladder.

NURSING DIAGNOSIS

High risk for ineffective breathing pattern related to location of surgical incision and pain

DESIRED PATIENT OUTCOME

The patient will maintain an effective breathing pattern

Outcome measurement criteria

- ☐ Respiratory rate of 12 to 20 breaths/minute
- ☐ Absence of shallow breathing
- ☐ Absence of adventitious lung sounds
- ☐ Oxygen saturation above 95% or at baseline value
- ☐ Demonstration of correct technique for diaphragmatic breathing
- ☐ Demonstration of correct use of incentive spirometer

Key interventions

- Assess respiratory status every 4 hours, observing respiratory rate and depth.
- Check for adventitious breath sounds, especially in right bases, every 4 hours.
- Assist with turning and repositioning every 2 hours.
- Instruct the patient to splint incision with pillow when deep breathing and coughing.
- Teach correct technique for diaphragmatic breathing to increase lung expansion.

- Teach the patient how to use incentive spirometer, and encourage its use every 2 hours.
- Monitor pulse oximetry values during each shift. Report significant changes.
- Administer pain medication before breathing exercises and ambulation, as prescribed.

NURSING DIAGNOSIS

High risk for fluid volume deficit related to possible hemorrhage secondary to decreased vitamin K absorption

DESIRED PATIENT OUTCOME

The patient will maintain an adequate fluid balance

Outcome measurement criteria

☐ Balanced fluid intake and output

☐ Absence of bleeding from gums, nose, and injection sites

☐ Absence of blood in urine and stool

☐ Prothrombin time (PT) within normal range

☐ Blood pressure within normal range

Key interventions

- Measure and record fluid intake and output.
- Monitor vital signs for decreasing blood pressure, weak pulse, and orthostatic changes, which indicate fluid loss.
- Instruct the patient to report bleeding from gums and nose and blood in urine or stool.
- Use small-gauge needles when giving injections. Apply pressure to injection sites to prevent bleeding.
- Observe injection sites for prolonged bleeding.

- Monitor PT values and report significant changes to the physician.
- Administer vitamin K, as prescribed.

NURSING DIAGNOSIS

Altered nutrition: less than body requirements related to nothing-by-mouth status, nasogastric (NG) intubation, and altered lipid metabolism

DESIRED PATIENT OUTCOME

The patient will regain adequate nutritional intake

Outcome measurement criteria

- ☐ Balanced fluid intake and output
- ☐ Maintenance of adequate nutritional intake
- ☐ Maintenance of stable weight
- ☐ Demonstration of tolerance of prescribed diet
- ☐ Absence of need for NG suction
- ☐ Absence of nausea and vomiting
- ☐ Serum albumin and protein values within normal ranges

Key interventions

- Measure and record fluid intake and output.
- Monitor nutritional intake. Maintain calorie count, if necessary.
- Weigh the patient daily and record results.
- Observe for nausea and vomiting. Intervene promptly, as needed.
- Maintain I.V. fluid therapy, as ordered, until the patient can tolerate oral fluids.
- Monitor output from NG tube and T tube.

- Remove NG tube, as ordered, once peristalsis returns.
- Monitor for return of peristalsis.
- Clamp T tube during meals.
- Offer clear liquids initially and then advance to low-fat, regular diet as tolerated.
- Provide small, frequent feedings to minimize abdominal distention.
- Monitor serum protein and albumin values. Report significant changes to the physician.
- Instruct the patient to avoid fatty foods for up to 6 months after discharge.

NURSING DIAGNOSIS

High risk for infection related to surgical tissue trauma and drainage tubes

DESIRED PATIENT OUTCOME

The patient will remain free of infection

Outcome measurement criteria

- ☐ Oral temperature at or below 99.0° F (37.2° C)
- ☐ White blood cell (WBC) count within normal range
- ☐ Absence of redness, swelling, warmth, and purulent drainage at incision site
- ☐ Absence of pain, nausea, and vomiting

Key interventions

- Measure oral temperature every 4 hours.
- Observe for chills, flushing, and diaphoresis.
- Monitor WBC count. Report significant changes to the physician.
- Assess wound for signs of infection during each shift.

- Monitor for signs and symptoms of T-tube obstruction, including pain in right upper abdominal quadrant, bile drainage around tube, jaundice, and dark yellow urine.
- Teach the patient and family how to care for T tube and insertion site after discharge.
- Teach the patient how to recognize signs and symptoms of infection. Emphasize importance of reporting these to the primary health care practitioner.

Cirrhosis

Chronic, degenerative liver disease characterized by widespread liver fibrosis, parenchymal degeneration, and fatty infiltration of lobules.

NURSING DIAGNOSIS

Ineffective breathing pattern related to decreased lung expansion secondary to ascites

DESIRED PATIENT OUTCOME

The patient will regain an effective breathing pattern

Outcome measurement criteria

☐ Respiratory rate of 12 to 20 breaths/minute

☐ Absence of shallow breathing

☐ Absence of adventitious lung sounds

☐ Absence of pneumonia and atelectasis

☐ Verbalization of more comfortable breathing

☐ Arterial blood gas (ABG) values within normal ranges

☐ Oxygen saturation above 95%

☐ Decreasing abdominal girth

Key interventions

- Assess respiratory status every 4 hours. Stay alert for difficulty breathing and adventitious lung sounds, such as crackles, rhonchi, and wheezes.
- Monitor vital signs frequently.
- Maintain the patient in high Fowler's position to promote breathing.

- Measure abdominal girth at same location daily, and record results.
- Reposition the patient frequently to increase comfort.
- Assist with activity and ambulation if the patient is short of breath.
- Monitor ABG and pulse oximetry values. Report significant changes to the physician.

NURSING DIAGNOSIS

Altered thought processes related to increased serum ammonia level secondary to liver disease

DESIRED PATIENT OUTCOME

The patient will regain orientation to person, place, and time

Outcome measurement criteria

☐ Serum ammonia level within normal range

☐ Absence of lethargy, confusion, and drowsiness

☐ Absence of signs and symptoms of physical injury

☐ Orientation to person, place, and time

Key interventions

- Assess the patient for alterations in level of consciousness and behavior.
- Observe for irritability, drowsiness, lethargy, and confusion. Notify the physician of significant findings.
- Reorient the patient, as needed.
- Take measures to prevent injury, such as keeping side rails up, maintaining bed in low position, keeping call bell within the patient's reach, and checking the patient frequently.

- Monitor serum ammonia levels. Report significant changes to the physician.
- Explain the patient's personality and behavior changes to the family to help decrease fear.

NURSING DIAGNOSIS

Altered nutrition: less than body requirements related to decreased oral intake

DESIRED PATIENT OUTCOME

The patient will regain adequate nutritional intake

Outcome measurement criteria

- ☐ Absence of nausea, vomiting, and indigestion
- ☐ Consumption of at least 50% of meals and snacks
- ☐ Maintenance of adequate weight and muscle mass
- ☐ Absence of evidence of alcohol consumption

Key interventions

- Assess the patient's nutritional status.
- Discuss the patient's normal eating patterns and food preferences.
- Offer small, frequent feedings throughout day. Provide foods that are high in calories, carbohydrates, and fats.
- Monitor for nausea, vomiting, and indigestion. Intervene to provide relief, as needed.
- Weigh the patient daily and record results.
- Monitor fluid intake and output.
- Monitor nutritional intake. Maintain calorie count, if necessary.

- Consult the dietitian regarding nutrition teaching. Include the family in teaching sessions whenever possible.

NURSING DIAGNOSIS

Fluid volume deficit related to diuretic therapy and fluid shifts secondary to liver disease

DESIRED PATIENT OUTCOME

The patient will regain an adequate fluid balance

Outcome measurement criteria

☐ Balanced fluid intake and output

☐ Decreasing abdominal girth

☐ Diminishing peripheral edema

☐ Serum electrolyte values within normal ranges

Key interventions

- Measure and record fluid intake and output.
- Measure abdominal girth in same location daily, and record results.
- Weigh the patient daily, preferably at same time each day. Consider weight loss of 1 to 1.5 lb/day acceptable, until the patient reaches baseline weight.
- Observe for edema in dependent areas, such as feet and legs. Observe for sacral edema if the patient is on bed rest.
- Administer diuretics, as prescribed, and document the patient's response.
- Monitor serum and urine electrolyte values. Report significant changes to the physician.

NURSING DIAGNOSIS

Ineffective family coping: compromised related to progressive nature of disease

DESIRED PATIENT OUTCOME

The family will demonstrate positive coping skills

Outcome measurement criteria

- ☐ Verbalization of need for additional information
- ☐ Verbalization of concerns and feelings about disease
- ☐ Discussion of changing roles within the family
- ☐ Verbalization of knowledge of appropriate support systems and support people
- ☐ Verbalization of decreased anxiety
- ☐ Demonstration of positive coping skills

Key interventions

- Observe patient-family interaction and family dynamics.
- Provide opportunities for the family to discuss concerns and feelings.
- Assess the family's and patient's knowledge. Provide information about the patient's disease, as needed.
- Discuss positive coping mechanisms used successfully by family members to deal with difficult situations in past. Help them adapt these mechanisms to present situation.
- Help family members recognize role changes needed to maintain the family during the patient's illness.
- Discuss role of alcoholism in disease. Encourage the family to attend community support groups and education classes to develop additional coping skills.

- Consult the social services department for additional counseling and referral.

NURSING DIAGNOSIS

High risk for injury related to alcohol withdrawal

DESIRED PATIENT OUTCOME

The patient will remain free of injury during hospitalization

Outcome measurement criteria

☐ Absence of signs and symptoms of physical injury

☐ Vital signs within normal ranges

☐ Decrease in agitation and tremors

☐ Absence of seizures

☐ Absence of hallucinations and delusions

☐ Absence of suicidal behavior

☐ Absence of evidence of alcohol consumption

Key interventions

- Assess the patient's normal alcohol consumption pattern. Determine time, type, and amount of last alcohol consumption. Find out if the patient uses other chemical substances.
- Monitor for signs and symptoms of alcohol withdrawal, such as tremors, hyperactivity, agitation, disorientation, delusions, attention or memory impairment, and elevations in blood pressure, heart rate, and respirations.
- Limit number of caregivers to prevent overstimulation.
- Maintain quiet environment.

- Keep room adequately lit, especially at night, to minimize hallucinations.
- Administer anxiolytic agents, as prescribed, to prevent serious alcohol withdrawal symptoms, such as delirium tremens and seizures. Be aware that the chronic alcoholic requires higher anxiolytic doses to achieve desired result.
- Evaluate effectiveness of prescribed medication.
- Notify the physician of significant changes in the patient's behavior.
- Explain all procedures, medications, and treatments to the patient and family to help decrease anxiety.
- Take measures to prevent injury, such as keeping side rails up, keeping bed in low position, and applying restraints, if needed and ordered.
- Monitor the patient every 10 minutes, or according to facility policy, if leather restraints are used. Pad restraints to prevent skin injury. Keep restraint key readily available in case of emergency. Release restraints one at a time to ensure adequate circulation.
- Protect and support the patient's head and establish open airway if seizure occurs.

Esophagitis and gastroenteritis

Esophagitis is an inflammation of mucosal lining of esophagus caused by gastric reflux, irritation, or infection; gastroenteritis is an inflammation of stomach and intestines caused by such GI conditions as bacterial or viral infection, bacterial endotoxins, and chemical toxins.

NURSING DIAGNOSIS

Pain related to inflammation

DESIRED PATIENT OUTCOME

The patient will experience relief from pain

Outcome measurement criteria

☐ Verbalization of adequate pain relief

☐ Vital signs within normal ranges

☐ Relaxed facial expression and muscle tone

☐ Use of stress-reduction techniques as part of daily routine

Key interventions

- Ask the patient to describe pain, including its severity, duration, frequency, location, and relation to activities or ingestion of certain foods.
- Check for nonverbal signs of pain.
- Monitor vital signs.
- Encourage the patient to request pain medication before pain becomes severe.
- Assess for belching, abdominal cramps, and diarrhea.

- Administer antispasmodic, antiemetic, and antidiarrheal medications, as prescribed and needed, to ease GI discomfort.
- Monitor and document effectiveness of prescribed medication.
- Help the patient identify stressors and minimize stress. Explain relation between stress and illness.
- Promote adequate rest and stress reduction.
- Teach the patient how to perform relaxation techniques.
- Instruct the patient to avoid eating for 2 to 3 hours before going to bed, to avoid smoking cigarettes, and to elevate head of bed for comfort while sleeping.

NURSING DIAGNOSIS

Altered nutrition: less than body requirements related to nausea, vomiting, and painful swallowing

DESIRED PATIENT OUTCOME

The patient will regain adequate nutritional intake

Outcome measurement criteria

- ☐ Verbalization of relief from nausea and vomiting
- ☐ Verbalization of absence of pain when swallowing
- ☐ Adequate fluid intake and output
- ☐ Maintenance of adequate weight

Key interventions

- Monitor fluid intake and output.
- Weigh the patient daily.
- Monitor for nausea, vomiting, and difficulty swallowing.

- Administer antiemetics, as prescribed and needed, and document the patient's response.
- Provide viscous lidocaine mouthwash, as needed, to reduce throat discomfort.
- Inspect inside of mouth for sores.
- Provide soft, bland foods in small, frequent feedings.
- Provide liquid nutritional supplements, as ordered.
- Advise the patient to avoid spicy foods, alcohol, and beverages and foods containing caffeine, which may worsen pain by increasing hydrochloric acid secretion.

NURSING DIAGNOSIS

High risk for fluid volume deficit related to diarrhea and vomiting secondary to GI inflammation

DESIRED PATIENT OUTCOME

The patient will maintain an adequate fluid balance

Outcome measurement criteria

☐ Balanced fluid intake and output

☐ Adequate skin turgor

☐ Absence of excessive thirst

☐ Absence of vomiting and diarrhea

☐ Vital signs within normal ranges

☐ Serum electrolyte levels within normal ranges

Key interventions

- Monitor vital signs every 4 hours.
- Observe for signs and symptoms of dehydration, including poor skin turgor, dry skin, excessive thirst, and weight loss.

- Monitor serum electrolyte levels and report significant changes to the physician.
- Provide preferred fluids frequently. Encourage the family to offer fluids during visits.
- Measure and record fluid intake and output.
- Administer antidiarrheal and antiemetic medications, as prescribed, and document their effectiveness.

NURSING DIAGNOSIS

High risk for altered body temperature related to inflammation secondary to invading organism

DESIRED PATIENT OUTCOME

The patient will maintain body temperature within the normal range

Outcome measurement criteria

☐ Oral temperature at or below 99.0° F (37.2° C)

☐ Absence of chills, flushing, and diaphoresis

☐ Cool, dry skin

Key interventions

- Measure oral temperature at least every 4 hours.
- Administer antipyretic agents, as prescribed.
- Observe for chills, diaphoresis, flushing, and hot, excessively dry skin.
- Keep room at temperature that is comfortable for the patient.
- Offer fluids frequently.
- Remove excess bed linens and clothing to promote heat loss.

NURSING DIAGNOSIS

Diarrhea related to invading organism

DESIRED PATIENT OUTCOME

The patient will regain normal bowel function

Outcome measurement criteria

- ☐ Absence of diarrhea
- ☐ Absence of abdominal cramps
- ☐ Negative stool cultures

Key interventions

- Measure liquid stools to determine rate of fluid loss.
- Obtain stool specimen for culture and send to laboratory. If specimen cannot be delivered immediately, call laboratory to determine if it should be refrigerated.
- Provide adequate bathroom ventilation and privacy to decrease the patient's embarrassment regarding odors.
- Administer antidiarrheal medication, as prescribed.
- Clean and lubricate perianal area to help prevent skin breakdown.
- Encourage the patient to wash hands scrupulously after using toilet to prevent spread of infection.

Gastrointestinal hemorrhage

Bleeding within GI tract caused by ulcer disease, tumor, or varices; more common and more serious in upper than lower GI tract.

NURSING DIAGNOSIS

Fluid volume deficit related to blood loss

DESIRED PATIENT OUTCOME

The patient will regain an adequate fluid balance

Outcome measurement criteria

☐ Vital signs within normal ranges

☐ Adequate skin turgor

☐ Absence of vomiting and diarrhea

☐ Absence of excessive thirst

☐ Decrease in amount of dark, tarry stools

☐ Absence of bloody or coffee-ground-like emesis

☐ Urine output of at least 60 ml/hour

☐ Hemoglobin and hematocrit values within normal ranges

Key interventions

- Monitor vital signs every 4 hours. Stay alert for decreasing blood pressure, pallor, and weak, thready pulse, which suggest hypovolemic shock.
- Assess for signs and symptoms of dehydration, including poor skin turgor, dry skin, excessive thirst, and weight loss.

- Monitor hemoglobin and hematocrit values. Report significant changes to the physician.
- Maintain I.V. fluids, as prescribed.
- Administer blood products, as prescribed.
- Insert nasogastric (NG) tube, as ordered, and perform gastric lavage with iced or room-temperature saline solution to stop bleeding.
- Maintain accurate record of fluid intake and output.
- Inspect all output, including stools, emesis, and NG drainage. Test drainage for occult blood. Report frank bleeding to the physician immediately.
- Administer vitamin K, as prescribed.
- Prepare the patient for transfer to intensive care unit, if necessary.

NURSING DIAGNOSIS

Fatigue related to decreased oxygen supply secondary to blood loss

DESIRED PATIENT OUTCOME

The patient will express a sense of reduced fatigue

Outcome measurement criteria

- ☐ Verbalization of decreasing fatigue and increasing energy
- ☐ Participation in basic self-care
- ☐ Absence of orthostatic hypotension
- ☐ Demonstration of ability to move from bed to chair or commode
- ☐ Demonstration of ability to ambulate short distances with assistance

- ☐ Verbalization of ability to sleep uninterrupted for 3- to 4-hour periods

Key interventions

- Maintain the patient on bed rest during active bleeding.
- Schedule rest periods between procedures and care activities.
- Provide supplemental oxygen, as prescribed and needed.
- Monitor for signs and symptoms of decreased circulating blood volume, such as shortness of breath, pallor, reduced blood pressure, lethargy, and confusion.
- Provide adequate parenteral nutrition and supplements, as ordered.
- Allow for periods of uninterrupted sleep. Promote sleep by providing warm bath, back rub, or sedative, if ordered.
- Encourage gradual participation in self-care. Assist the patient, as needed.
- Advise the patient to change position slowly to avoid orthostatic hypotension, such as by sitting on side of bed and dangling legs before moving to chair or commode.

NURSING DIAGNOSIS

Fear related to bleeding and unpredictable course of illness

DESIRED PATIENT OUTCOME

The patient will express decreased fear

Outcome measurement criteria

- ☐ Communication of fears to staff
- ☐ Verbalization of decreased fear

☐ Verbalization of understanding of diagnostic procedures and treatments

☐ Verbalization of ability to get adequate sleep

Key interventions

- Encourage the patient to discuss fears.
- Determine cause of fear and attempt to alleviate it.
- Reassure the patient that fear is normal response to situation.
- Maintain calm, accepting manner.
- Explain all diagnostic procedures and treatments to the patient and family. Stay with the patient during procedures.
- Observe for signs and symptoms of increasing fear and anxiety, and intervene promptly.

Gastrointestinal surgery

Surgical procedure involving GI tract, such as appendectomy, colectomy, or bowel resection.

NURSING DIAGNOSIS

Pain related to surgery, manipulation of GI tract, and flatulence

DESIRED PATIENT OUTCOME

The patient will experience relief from pain

Outcome measurement criteria

☐ Verbalization of decreased pain

☐ Vital signs within normal ranges

☐ Relaxed facial expression and muscle tone

☐ Participation in self-care

Key interventions

- Ask the patient to describe nature, location, and severity of pain.
- Determine effects of pain on the patient's appetite, mental state, and activity.
- Explain principles of postoperative pain management, including meaning of *p.r.n.*
- Discuss use of patient-controlled analgesia (PCA), if applicable. Teach the patient how to use PCA pump. Observe return demonstration.
- Reassure the patient and family that postoperative narcotic addiction is rare.

- Encourage the patient to request pain medication before pain becomes severe.
- Administer analgesics before activities, as prescribed.
- Evaluate effectiveness of pain medication. Monitor for adverse narcotic effects, especially respiratory depression.
- Switch to oral analgesics, as prescribed, when pain decreases and the patient can tolerate oral intake.
- Explain that ambulation helps relieve flatulence.
- Consult the physician and clinical pharmacist if pain management is ineffective.

NURSING DIAGNOSIS

Ineffective breathing pattern related to narcotics and abdominal pain

DESIRED PATIENT OUTCOME

The patient will regain an effective breathing pattern

Outcome measurement criteria

☐ Respiratory rate of 12 to 20 breaths/minute

☐ Absence of adventitious lung sounds

☐ Arterial blood gas (ABG) and pulse oximetry values within normal ranges

☐ Normal skin color

☐ Absence of pneumonia and atelectasis

☐ Verbalization of increasing comfort in breathing

☐ Demonstration of correct techniques for coughing, deep breathing, splinting, and using incentive spirometer

Key interventions

- Assess respiratory status every 4 hours, noting adventitious lung sounds.
- Observe for splinting, shallow breathing, and dyspnea.
- Monitor vital signs frequently.
- Monitor ABG and pulse oximetry values. Report significant changes to the physician.
- Encourage the patient to turn, cough, and perform deep-breathing every 2 hours.
- Teach the patient how to splint incision. Observe return demonstration.
- Assist with activities of daily living and early ambulation, as needed.

NURSING DIAGNOSIS

High risk for infection related to tissue trauma and increased risk of contamination secondary to intestinal surgery

DESIRED PATIENT OUTCOME

The patient will remain free of infection

Outcome measurement criteria

☐ Oral temperature at or below 99.0° F (37.2° C)

☐ White blood cell (WBC) count within normal range

☐ Absence of erythema, purulent drainage, and tenderness at incision site

☐ Approximation of wound edges

☐ Negative blood and wound cultures

Key interventions

- Measure oral temperature at least every 4 hours.

- Observe for chills, diaphoresis, and changes in vital signs.
- Monitor WBC count for increases that suggest infection, and report these to the physician.
- Assess wound for warmth, redness, drainage, tenderness, and odor during each shift.
- Obtain blood or wound cultures, as needed, and monitor results.
- Consult the infection control practitioner, as needed.

NURSING DIAGNOSIS

Constipation related to decreased GI motility secondary to surgery

DESIRED PATIENT OUTCOME

The patient will regain normal bowel function

Outcome measurement criteria

☐ Presence of bowel sounds

☐ Adequate fluid intake

☐ Resumption of bowel movements

☐ Absence of constipation

☐ Absence of abdominal distention

Key interventions

- Assess abdomen every 4 hours. Listen for bowel sounds in all quadrants.
- Observe for abdominal distention and tension on suture line.
- Monitor for first postoperative bowel movement.
- Notify the physician if bowel sounds do not resume or if bowel movement does not occur by specified time.

- Assess dietary intake, and advance diet as tolerated.
- Offer fluids to promote bowel function.
- Evaluate color, consistency, frequency, and amount of stools.
- Encourage early ambulation to decrease flatulence.

NURSING DIAGNOSIS

Impaired skin integrity related to inflammation and excessive wound drainage

DESIRED PATIENT OUTCOME

The patient will maintain intact skin

Outcome measurement criteria

- ☐ Absence of skin breakdown and drainage around wound
- ☐ Approximation of wound edges
- ☐ Lack of pressure from drainage tube at tube insertion site

Key interventions

- Assess wound for signs of infection.
- Monitor wound dressing for excessive drainage. Consider using wound pouching system if drainage is excessive.
- Use wafer or Montgomery straps instead of taping dressing to skin.
- Change wound dressing frequently to protect skin.
- Tape tubes securely and protect surrounding skin to help prevent pulling of tubes.
- Observe nares for pressure from nasogastric tube.

- Consult the enterostomal therapist for postoperative management recommendations.

NURSING DIAGNOSIS

High risk for impaired home maintenance management related to lack of information about follow-up care

DESIRED PATIENT OUTCOME

The patient or family members will verbalize understanding of plan to manage the patient at home

Outcome measurement criteria

☐ Demonstration of correct wound care technique

☐ Verbalization of activity guidelines and restrictions

☐ Demonstration of correct technique for care of drainage tubes

☐ Verbalization of prescribed medication regimen

☐ Verbalization of conditions to report to the primary health care practitioner

☐ Verbalization of available community and home care resources

Key interventions

- Teach the patient and family correct techniques for wound and drainage tube care. Observe several return demonstrations to verify mastery.
- Discuss activity guidelines and restrictions, including importance of walking regularly, getting adequate rest, and avoiding heavy lifting for 6 to 8 weeks.
- Review names, purposes, dosages, administration routes, and common adverse effects of all prescribed medications.

- Advise the patient to splint incision when coughing or sneezing.
- Instruct the patient to report redness, pain, or drainage at incision site.
- Provide information on home care resources, if necessary.
- Consult the social services department for home care assistance if the patient cannot care for self at home.

Hepatitis

Inflammation of liver resulting from such conditions as viral or bacterial infection, alcohol, drugs, and transfusion of incompatible blood; disease course and outcome vary with cause.

NURSING DIAGNOSIS

Altered protection related to liver infection and invading organism

DESIRED PATIENT OUTCOME

The patient will remain free of infection

Outcome measurement criteria

- ☐ Oral temperature at or below 99.0° F (37.2° C)
- ☐ White blood cell (WBC) count within normal range
- ☐ Absence of chills, diaphoresis, and flushing
- ☐ Demonstration of ability to maintain isolation precautions
- ☐ Absence of pain in right upper abdominal quadrant
- ☐ Results of liver function tests within acceptable range for disease stage

Key interventions

- Monitor vital signs every 4 hours. Check for elevated temperature, pain, diaphoresis, and chills.
- Administer antipyretics, as prescribed and needed.
- Provide comfort measures to reduce fever, as needed.
- Monitor WBC and results of liver function tests. Report significant changes to the physician.

- Teach the patient and family about disease course and possible infection spread. Obtain information about patient contacts who may need prophylaxis.
- Consult the infection control practitioner about possible need for isolation. Follow infection control and isolation procedures to help prevent infection spread.

NURSING DIAGNOSIS

Altered nutrition: less than body requirements related to nausea, vomiting, and anorexia

DESIRED PATIENT OUTCOME

The patient will regain adequate nutritional intake

Outcome measurement criteria

- ☐ Adequate caloric intake
- ☐ Maintenance of stable weight
- ☐ Absence of nausea and vomiting
- ☐ Verbalization of adequate appetite

Key interventions

- Determine the patient's normal eating patterns and food preferences.
- Offer small, frequent meals throughout day if the patient can tolerate oral intake. Serve largest meal in morning because anorexia worsens as day progresses. Provide high-carbohydrate, low-fat foods to aid digestion.
- Administer parenteral nutrition, if prescribed and needed.
- Monitor the patient's nutritional status.
- Monitor for nausea and vomiting. Intervene as needed, such as by giving hard candy to relieve nausea.

- Weigh the patient daily and record results.
- Monitor fluid intake and output.
- Maintain calorie count, if necessary.
- Ask the dietitian to provide assistance with nutrition teaching. Include the family in teaching sessions whenever possible.

NURSING DIAGNOSIS

Activity intolerance related to fatigue and weakness

DESIRED PATIENT OUTCOME

The patient will tolerate a gradual increase in activity

Outcome measurement criteria

- ☐ Demonstration of increasing ability to perform self-care independently
- ☐ Demonstration of independent ambulation
- ☐ Verbalization of decreased fatigue
- ☐ Absence of shortness of breath
- ☐ Absence of dizziness and vertigo
- ☐ Vital signs within normal ranges

Key interventions

- Monitor the patient's physiologic response to activity.
- Monitor vital signs. Observe for orthostatic changes with activity.
- Provide supplemental oxygen, if needed and prescribed.
- Schedule rest periods between activities.
- Instruct the patient to report vertigo, shortness of breath, and other signs of fatigue during activity.

- Assist with self-care, as needed. Encourage the patient to participate to tolerance level.

NURSING DIAGNOSIS

Knowledge deficit related to disease transmission and recurrence

DESIRED PATIENT OUTCOME

The patient will verbalize an understanding of disease transmission and follow-up care

Outcome measurement criteria

- ☐ Verbalization of understanding of disease process and transmission
- ☐ Verbalization of understanding of appropriate body fluid precautions
- ☐ Demonstration of scrupulous personal hygiene practices
- ☐ Verbalization of activities to avoid
- ☐ Verbalization of importance of follow-up care

Key interventions

- Teach the patient about relevant type of hepatitis, and review expected disease course. Ask for return explanation.
- Explain that hepatitis is transmitted through fecal-oral route, contaminated food or water, and direct or indirect contact with infected body fluids, including blood, saliva, and semen.
- Inform family members of need for hepatitis vaccination.
- Instruct the patient with hepatitis A not to share utensils or toothbrushes and not to prepare food for others when symptomatic.

- Teach the patient to avoid sexual activity during acute disease phase. Caution the patient with hepatitis B to refrain from sexual activity until blood studies are negative or until the partner has been vaccinated.
- Emphasize need for scrupulous personal hygiene.
- Instruct the patient to avoid alcohol, sedatives, and aspirin during acute disease phase.
- Emphasize importance of follow-up liver function tests until results are negative.

Pancreatitis

Acute or chronic inflammation of pancreas usually caused by biliary tract disease, such as from alcohol abuse or infection.

NURSING DIAGNOSIS

Altered nutrition: less than body requirements related to malabsorption

DESIRED PATIENT OUTCOME

The patient will regain adequate nutritional intake

Outcome measurement criteria

- ☐ Maintenance of stable weight
- ☐ Absence of diarrhea and steatorrhea
- ☐ Absence of nausea and vomiting
- ☐ Consumption of at least 50% of meals
- ☐ Balanced fluid intake and output
- ☐ Monitor nutritional intake. Maintain calorie count, if necessary.
- ☐ Serum and urine glucose levels within normal ranges
- ☐ Demonstration of correct technique for self-administering parenteral nutrition

Key interventions

- Assess abdomen at least every 4 hours. Note mild distention and tenderness and absent bowel sounds.
- Consult the nutritionist to determine the patient's dietary needs and most appropriate way to meet them.
- Withhold oral intake during acute disease episodes.

- Provide frequent mouth and nares care if nasogastric tube is in place.
- Provide small, frequent, high-protein, low-fat meals, if the patient can tolerate oral intake.
- Administer parenteral nutrition, if needed and prescribed.
- Teach the patient how to self-administer parenteral nutrition at home.
- Observe stools for diarrhea and steatorrhea.
- Monitor serum and urine glucose levels for evidence of transient hyperglycemia, a potential complication of acute pancreatitis.
- Instruct the patient to avoid coffee, spicy foods, and alcohol, which stimulate hydrochloric acid secretion.

NURSING DIAGNOSIS

Pain related to inflammation

DESIRED PATIENT OUTCOME

The patient will experience relief from pain

Outcome measurement criteria

☐ Verbalization of decreased pain

☐ Vital signs within normal ranges

☐ Relaxed facial expression and muscle tone

☐ Verbalization of ability to get adequate sleep

Key interventions

- Ask the patient to describe nature, location, and severity of pain. Be aware that pancreatic pain usually is epigastric, steady, dull, and boring and worsens when the patient is supine.

- Help the patient find comfortable sitting and forward-leaning positions.
- Administer pain medication, as prescribed, before activities and care procedures.
- Encourage the patient to request pain medication before pain becomes severe.
- Evaluate and document effectiveness of pain medication.

NURSING DIAGNOSIS

High risk for fluid volume deficit related to nausea, vomiting, and fluid shifts

DESIRED PATIENT OUTCOME

The patient will maintain an adequate fluid balance

Outcome measurement criteria

☐ Adequate fluid intake

☐ Balanced fluid intake and output

☐ Absence of nausea and vomiting

☐ Normal skin turgor

☐ Intact oral mucous membranes

☐ Vital signs within normal ranges

☐ Serum electrolyte levels within normal ranges

☐ Hemoglobin and hematocrit values within normal ranges

Key interventions

- Assess for signs and symptoms of dehydration, including poor skin turgor, dry mucous membranes, thirst, concentrated urine, and low blood pressure.
- Measure and record fluid intake and output.

- Weigh the patient daily and record results.
- Monitor vital signs every 4 hours.
- Monitor hemoglobin, hematocrit, and serum electrolyte values. Notify the physician of significant changes.
- Administer I.V. fluids and fluid expanders, as prescribed.
- Offer preferred beverages frequently, unless the patient can receive nothing by mouth. Advise the patient to avoid coffee because this may worsen pain by increasing hydrochloric acid secretion.

NURSING DIAGNOSIS

High risk for ineffective management of therapeutic regimen related to lack of information and complex nature of treatment

DESIRED PATIENT OUTCOME

The patient will develop a plan for integrating the therapeutic regimen into daily life

Outcome measurement criteria

- ☐ Verbalization of importance of participating in alcohol rehabilitation program, if applicable
- ☐ Verbalization of understanding of disease process and treatment
- ☐ Description of strategies to prevent disease recurrence
- ☐ Identification of available community resources and support groups
- ☐ Demonstration of correct technique for self-administering parenteral nutrition, if applicable

Key interventions

- Explain disease process and possible causes of disease to the patient and family.
- Ask the dietitian to provide education about low-fat, high-protein, high-carbohydrate diet.
- Emphasize importance of avoiding alcohol and stopping smoking because alcohol and smoking exacerbate pancreatitis.
- Teach the patient and family about hyperglycemia as potential complication. Review signs and symptoms of hyperglycemia, and explain role of insulin therapy.
- Encourage the family to ask questions, and clarify misconceptions.
- Teach the patient and family about home parenteral nutrition.
- Provide information about community resources and support groups.
- Contact home health agency or hospital home care department for assistance and follow-up.

Ulcer disease

Abnormal condition characterized by ulceration of gastric or duodenal mucosa caused by increased hydrochloric acid secretion (such as from stress, hereditary factors, medications, or chemical exposure).

NURSING DIAGNOSIS

Pain related to GI mucosal irritation

DESIRED PATIENT OUTCOME

The patient will experience relief from pain

Outcome measurement criteria

- ☐ Verbalization of decreased pain
- ☐ Vital signs within normal ranges
- ☐ Verbalization of absence of heartburn
- ☐ Relaxed facial expression
- ☐ Verbalization of ability to get adequate sleep

Key interventions

- Assess nature and location of pain and effectiveness of antacids in relieving pain.
- Stay alert for sudden onset of severe pain, which suggests perforation.
- Monitor gastric pH, as indicated.
- Administer pain medication and antacids, as prescribed.
- Observe for signs and symptoms of complications, including rigid abdomen, referred shoulder pain, dizziness, decreased blood pressure, and loss of antacid relief.

NURSING DIAGNOSIS

High risk for fluid volume deficit related to blood loss secondary to GI hemorrhage

DESIRED PATIENT OUTCOME

The patient will maintain an adequate fluid balance

Outcome measurement criteria

- ☐ Balanced fluid intake and output
- ☐ Hemoglobin and hematocrit values within normal ranges
- ☐ Vital signs within normal ranges
- ☐ Absence of signs and symptoms of active bleeding
- ☐ Absence of occult blood in emesis and stools

Key interventions

- Assess vital signs every 4 hours or more often if indicated. Observe for decreased blood pressure and weak, thready pulse.
- Measure and record fluid intake and output.
- Test emesis and stools for occult blood.
- Monitor hemoglobin and hematocrit values. Report significant changes to the physician.
- Administer I.V. fluids, as prescribed.
- Prepare the patient for endoscopy, if indicated.

NURSING DIAGNOSIS

Anxiety related to pain and stress

DESIRED PATIENT OUTCOME

The patient will demonstrate decreased anxiety

Outcome measurement criteria

- ☐ Verbalization of concerns and fears
- ☐ Discussion of stressors
- ☐ Demonstration of relaxation and stress-reduction techniques
- ☐ Verbalization of support systems
- ☐ Verbalization of decreased anxiety

Key interventions

- Encourage the patient to discuss concerns and fears.
- Assess for signs and symptoms of anxiety.
- Help identify stressors that may exacerbate ulcer disease.
- Discuss ways to modify behavior and habits to reduce stress.
- Provide diversional activities to reduce anxiety.
- Explain all procedures. Stay with the patient and provide reassurance during procedures to allay fears.
- Teach the patient how to perform deep breathing and progressive relaxation. Observe return demonstrations.
- Encourage the patient to perform relaxation exercises several times a day to reduce stress.
- Provide information on community classes, support groups, and counseling services that will be available after discharge.
- Discuss with the physician the possible need for psychological or psychiatric consultation, if the patient's anxiety is severe.

NURSING DIAGNOSIS

High risk for ineffective management of therapeutic regimen related to lack of information and maladaptive coping mechanisms

DESIRED PATIENT OUTCOME

The patient will express an intent to follow the prescribed therapeutic regimen after discharge

Outcome measurement criteria

- ☐ Verbalization of correct dosages of all prescribed medications
- ☐ Verbalization of foods, beverages, and over-the-counter (OTC) medications to avoid
- ☐ Demonstration of stress-reduction techniques
- ☐ Verbalization of strategies to prevent ulcer recurrence

Key interventions

- Discuss disease process and possible causes of disease with the patient and family.
- Explain prescribed medication regimen. Verify that the patient understands which medications to take before and after meals.
- Provide the patient with verbal and written instructions regarding illness management after discharge.
- Encourage the patient to avoid practices that exacerbate ulcers, including smoking cigarettes and ingesting alcohol, coffee, and salicylates (for example, aspirin). Provide list of OTC medications containing salicylates.
- Inform the patient that milk is not an antacid and should not be used interchangeably with antacids. Mention that milk ingestion increases gastric acid secretion.

- Provide instructions on dietary management during acute disease phase, such as avoiding spices, citrus juices, tea, coffee, and alcohol.
- Emphasize the need for stress reduction and provide list of appropriate community resources. Suggest counseling if the patient is under severe stress.
- Emphasize the importance of continuing treatment even after symptoms subside.

Cerebrovascular accident (CVA)

Occlusion of cerebral blood vessels by cerebrovascular hemorrhage or embolus, resulting in ischemia to areas of brain normally perfused by affected vessels.

NURSING DIAGNOSIS

Impaired physical mobility related to motor deficit secondary to CVA

DESIRED PATIENT OUTCOME

The patient will demonstrate optimal mobility

Outcome measurement criteria

- ☐ Absence of contractures
- ☐ Demonstration of ability to move arms and legs within physiologic limitations
- ☐ Participation in activities of daily living within physiologic limitations
- ☐ Demonstration of correct technique for range-of-motion (ROM) exercises and use of assistive devices
- ☐ Absence of complications of immobility, such as pneumonia, venous stasis, thrombus, and skin breakdown

Key interventions

- Assess the patient's functional ability on admission, and monitor for changes during every shift.
- Turn and reposition the patient every 2 hours.

- Perform ROM exercises every 4 hours.
- Encourage the patient and family to participate in exercise regimen.
- Maintain proper body alignment using pillows, towel rolls, splints, and high-top sneakers.
- Elevate affected arms and legs on pillows, unless contraindicated.
- Use air mattress, foot board, trapeze bar, and other assistive devices, as needed.
- Teach the patient and family how to use assistive devices.
- Monitor for complications of immobility.
- Apply antiembolism stockings to help prevent venous stasis. Remove stockings for 1 hour each shift and then reapply.
- Provide assistance with progressive mobility as the patient's condition permits.
- Collaborate with the physical therapist to develop mobility plan. Reinforce instructions given by the physical therapist.
- Teach the patient to support affected side with unaffected side.
- Encourage participation in basic activities of daily living as soon as possible, using unaffected side.

NURSING DIAGNOSIS

Impaired verbal communication related to damage to cerebral speech center

DESIRED PATIENT OUTCOME

The patient will communicate needs effectively

Outcome measurement criteria

- ☐ Use of alternative communication method
- ☐ Consistent communication of needs to staff
- ☐ Demonstration of decreased frustration when communicating
- ☐ Evidence of satisfaction with chosen communication method

Key interventions

- Assess whether communication impairment is expressive, receptive, or both.
- Explain communication impairment to the patient and family. Encourage the family to support the patient.
- Allow the patient to choose from various alternative communication methods, such as paper and pencil, Magic Slate, picture board, and poster with common questions and phrases.
- Teach the patient how to use chosen communication method. Include the family in teaching sessions whenever possible.
- Provide positive reinforcement for communication attempts.
- Speak in short, simple phrases while standing within the patient's sight. Allow time for response.
- Speak in normal tone. Do not talk loudly or shout.
- Anticipate the patient's hygiene and toileting needs.
- Keep emergency call button within reach on the patient's unaffected side at all times.
- Reassure the patient that speech probably will improve gradually.
- Collaborate with the speech therapist to maximize the patient's ability to communicate.

NURSING DIAGNOSIS

High risk for impaired skin integrity related to immobility and inadequate nutrition

DESIRED PATIENT OUTCOME

The patient's skin will remain intact

Outcome measurement criteria

- ☐ Warm, dry skin
- ☐ Adequate skin turgor
- ☐ Normal skin color
- ☐ Strong peripheral pulses
- ☐ Adequate fluid intake and output
- ☐ Absence of redness, blistering, or edema (signs of impending or actual skin breakdown)
- ☐ Serum albumin and protein values within normal ranges

Key interventions

- Assess skin integrity at least every 4 hours by observing for redness, blistering, and edema, especially over bony prominences.
- Monitor skin turgor for evidence of dehydration.
- Palpate peripheral pulses.
- Assess skin temperature and capillary filling time.
- Document fluid intake and output carefully to evaluate fluid balance.
- Turn and reposition the patient with pillows every 2 hours.
- Perform passive or active ROM exercises on affected arms and legs.
- Encourage activity and ambulation to tolerance level.

- Keep skin clean and dry. Lubricate with lotion or oil.
- Use air mattress, heel and elbow pads, and other appropriate devices to help prevent skin breakdown.
- Use draw sheets to move the patient in bed.
- Monitor serum albumin and protein values to help assess nutritional status.
- Teach preventive skin care regimen to the patient and family. Observe return demonstration before discharge.

NURSING DIAGNOSIS

Altered cerebral tissue perfusion related to interrupted arterial flow

DESIRED PATIENT OUTCOME

The patient will exhibit signs of improved cerebral tissue perfusion

Outcome measurement criteria

☐ Improving level of consciousness (LOC)

☐ Orientation to person, place, and time

☐ Vital signs within normal ranges

☐ Arterial blood gas values within normal ranges

☐ Absence of marked behavioral problems

☐ Demonstration of ability to move arms and legs within physiologic limitations

Key interventions

- Assess neurologic status every 4 hours, including LOC, ability to move arms and legs, and pupillary response. Report subtle changes to the physician.

- Observe for behavioral changes, including increased agitation, belligerence, uncooperativeness, and unusual behavior toward family members.
- Remain calm if behavioral change occurs, and do not argue with the patient. Try to determine cause of behavioral change, and notify the physician.
- Elevate head of bed no more than 30 degrees. Maintain the patient's head in neutral alignment to promote perfusion.
- Maintain calm, quiet environment.
- Reorient the patient as needed. Place clock and calendar within the patient's sight.
- Encourage the family to discuss current events, family situations, and other topics of interest when visiting to help the patient stay alert and involved.
- Provide stool softeners to prevent straining at stool.
- Monitor blood pressure. Administer antihypertensives, as prescribed and needed.
- Monitor fluid balance and I.V. flow rates carefully to prevent fluid overload.

NURSING DIAGNOSIS

High risk for impaired swallowing related to neuromuscular impairment secondary to CVA

DESIRED PATIENT OUTCOME

The patient will demonstrate adequate swallowing

Outcome measurement criteria

- ☐ Absence of signs of aspiration
- ☐ Absence of coughing, choking, or food retention in mouth during meals
- ☐ Intact oral mucous membranes

☐ Adequate nutritional intake

☐ Demonstration by family members of correct techniques for feeding the patient, performing Heimlich maneuver, and suctioning

☐ Verbalization by family members of strategies to prevent aspiration

Key interventions

- Assess gag and cough reflexes before offering food or fluids.
- Assess ability to swallow saliva and then water.
- Elevate head of bed 90 degrees during meals.
- Instruct the patient to tilt head forward 45 degrees when eating or drinking to keep esophagus patent.
- Place food on unaffected side of mouth if paralysis is present.
- Advance diet from liquids to soft foods to solids, as tolerated.
- Inspect mouth frequently to check for retained food, and assess condition of mucous membranes.
- Keep suction apparatus at bedside at all times.
- Consult the speech therapist for swallowing evaluation, as needed.
- Teach the family correct techniques for Heimlich maneuver and suctioning.
- Instruct family members to help feed the patient. Be available to observe and supervise, as needed.

NURSING DIAGNOSIS

Self-care deficit: feeding, bathing, and/or toileting related to motor deficit secondary to CVA

DESIRED PATIENT OUTCOME

The patient will perform self-care activities with minimal assistance

Outcome measurement criteria

- ☐ Participation in self-care activities within physiologic limitations
- ☐ Verbalization of self-care needs
- ☐ Verbalization of concerns and frustrations
- ☐ Demonstration of decreased need for assistance with self-care activities
- ☐ Progressive improvement in motor and cognitive skills needed to perform self-care activities

Key interventions

- Assess the patient's functional abilities and limitations on admission, and monitor for changes daily.
- Discuss concerns and frustrations with the patient and family. Reassure them that frustration is normal response to situation.
- Anticipate hygiene and toileting needs to help decrease frustration. Offer bedpan or commode every 2 to 4 hours.
- Provide privacy during bathing and dressing. Do not rush the patient through these activities.
- Monitor fluid intake and output.
- Note episodes of incontinence.
- Keep call button within reach on the patient's unaffected side.
- Support independence. Encourage the patient to participate in daily care, and offer assistance as needed.
- Provide positive reinforcement for participation and progressive improvement in self-care.

- Maintain safe environment.
- Place the patient in high Fowler's position for meals.
- Assist during meals by placing food and utensils within the patient's reach, opening cartons, and cutting food, as necessary.
- Provide assistive devices to promote independence.
- Encourage the family to bring clothing that the patient can put on and remove easily.
- Teach the patient and family about home care and correct use of assistive devices that will be needed after discharge.
- Consult the occupational therapist for evaluation of the patient's ability to perform self-care.

Intracranial surgery

Surgical intervention to remove tumor, control bleeding, or relieve increased intracranial pressure (ICP).

NURSING DIAGNOSIS

Altered cerebral tissue perfusion related to inflammation

DESIRED PATIENT OUTCOME

The patient will exhibit signs of improved cerebral tissue perfusion

Outcome measurement criteria

- ☐ Absence of signs of deterioration in level of consciousness (LOC)
- ☐ Vital signs within normal ranges
- ☐ Evidence of alertness and orientation to person, place, and time
- ☐ Absence of seizures
- ☐ Demonstration of ability to move arms and legs within physiologic limitations

Key interventions

- Assess neurologic status at least every 4 hours, including LOC, motor function, and pupillary response. Report subtle changes to the physician.
- Monitor vital signs every 4 hours. Report sudden changes in blood pressure, pulse rate, and neurologic status.
- Orient the patient to person, place, and time, as needed.
- Place clock and calendar within the patient's sight.

- Observe for restlessness and seizures.
- Explain all procedures and treatments to the patient and family to decrease anxiety.
- Maintain calm, quiet environment.
- Maintain bed rest, with head of bed elevated 30 degrees.
- Avoid use of restraints and Valsalva maneuver.

NURSING DIAGNOSIS

Pain (headache) related to craniotomy incision and possible increase in ICP

DESIRED PATIENT OUTCOME

The patient will experience relief from pain

Outcome measurement criteria

- ☐ Verbalization of pain relief
- ☐ Vital signs within normal ranges
- ☐ Relaxed facial expression and muscle tone
- ☐ Absence of restlessness, nausea, and vomiting

Key interventions

- Assess for signs and symptoms of pain, including facial grimaces, restlessness, shallow breathing, muscle tension, and changes in vital signs.
- Observe for nausea, vomiting, pupillary changes, and deteriorating LOC, which suggest increasing ICP.
- Explain principles of postoperative pain control, including meaning of *p.r.n.*
- Monitor and document effectiveness of pain medication.
- Encourage the patient to request pain medication before pain becomes severe.

- Use patient-controlled analgesia (PCA), if appropriate. Teach the patient how to use PCA pump correctly.
- Implement additional pain control methods, such as relaxation, music, and guided imagery, as needed.
- Use appropriate interventions to decrease anxiety associated with pain. For instance, listen to the patient's concerns, explain the cause of pain, and reassure the patient that pain is normal and will subside. Explain that tension and anxiety may worsen pain. Teach deep-breathing techniques.
- Consult the physician and clinical pharmacist if pain management is ineffective.

NURSING DIAGNOSIS

High risk for ineffective airway clearance related to postoperative immobility and impaired cough reflex

DESIRED PATIENT OUTCOME

The patient will maintain a patent airway

Outcome measurement criteria

- ☐ Patent airway
- ☐ Decreased secretions
- ☐ Absence of adventitious lung sounds
- ☐ Absence of dyspnea and cyanosis
- ☐ Demonstration of effective cough
- ☐ Demonstration of ability to expectorate secretions
- ☐ Absence of signs and symptoms of aspiration

Key interventions

- Assess lung sounds and respiratory rate and effort every 4 hours. Document rhonchi, crackles, or wheezes.

- Suction airway, as needed.
- Keep head of bed elevated 45 degrees to promote breathing.
- Offer fluids to liquefy secretions, unless contraindicated by increased ICP. Withhold dairy products, which increase mucus viscosity.
- Reposition the patient every 2 hours to help mobilize secretions.
- Teach the patient effective coughing and deep-breathing techniques. Observe return demonstration.

NURSING DIAGNOSIS

High risk for trauma related to altered LOC and potential for seizures secondary to increased ICP

DESIRED PATIENT OUTCOME

The patient will remain free of injury

Outcome measurement criteria

☐ Absence of signs or symptoms of injury

☐ Evidence of alertness and orientation to person, place, and time

☐ Absence of seizures

Key interventions

- Implement seizure precautions, such as keeping bed in low position, padding side rails, and keeping oral airway and suction equipment at bedside.
- Monitor neurologic status and report significant changes to the physician.
- Keep call button within the patient's reach at all times.

- If seizure occurs, turn the patient onto side to keep airway open. Do not attempt to place anything in mouth during seizure. Provide privacy and stay with the patient.
- If seizure occurs when the patient is out of bed, ease the patient onto floor and support and protect the patient's head.
- Monitor vital signs and reorient the patient after seizure ends.
- Reassure the patient and family that patient safety will be maintained if seizures occur.

NURSING DIAGNOSIS

High risk for infection related to surgery

DESIRED PATIENT OUTCOME

The patient will remain free of infection

Outcome measurement criteria

- ☐ Oral temperature at or below 99.0° F (37.2° C)
- ☐ White blood cell (WBC) count within normal range
- ☐ Negative wound cultures
- ☐ Absence of erythema, tenderness, and purulent drainage at incision site
- ☐ Absence of stiff neck and other signs of meningitis

Key interventions

- Measure oral temperature at least every 4 hours.
- Assess wound for signs of infection during each shift.
- Monitor WBC count for increases that suggest infection. Report significant changes to the physician.

- Obtain wound cultures, as ordered, and report significant results.
- Observe for stitch abscess, which may precede wound infection.
- Monitor for signs and symptoms of meningitis, including severe headache, nausea, vomiting, stiff neck, photophobia, temperature elevation, decreased LOC, and seizures.
- Consult the infection control practitioner, as needed.

Meningitis

Inflammation or infection of meninges (membranes covering brain and spinal cord), usually of bacterial or viral origin.

NURSING DIAGNOSIS

High risk for infection related to inflammation secondary to invading organism

DESIRED PATIENT OUTCOME

The patient will remain free of infection

Outcome measurement criteria

☐ Oral temperature at or below 99.0° F (37.2° C)

☐ White blood cell count within normal range

☐ Absence of rash or ecchymosis

☐ Absence of Kernig's and Brudzinski's signs

☐ Demonstration of alertness and orientation

Key interventions

- Measure oral temperature at least every 4 hours.
- Inspect skin for rash and ecchymosis.
- Monitor neurologic status and cranial nerve function.
- Assess for Kernig's sign (pain or resistance when the knee is straightened after the leg is flexed at the hip and knee). Notify the physician if this sign is present.
- Assess for Brudzinski's sign (involuntary knee flexion when the neck is flexed passively). Notify the physician if this sign is present.
- Administer antibiotics, as prescribed, to achieve optimal blood drug levels.

- Explain course of illness and spread of infection to the patient and family.
- Obtain information about patient contacts who may require prophylactic treatment.
- Consult the infection control practitioner regarding possible need for isolation. Follow infection control and isolation procedures to prevent further spread of infection.

NURSING DIAGNOSIS

High risk for altered body temperature related to inflammation secondary to invading organism

DESIRED PATIENT OUTCOME

The patient will maintain body temperature within the normal range

Outcome measurement criteria

☐ Oral temperature at or below 99.0° F (37.2° C)

☐ Absence of chills, flushing, and diaphoresis

☐ Cool, dry skin

☐ Absence of seizures

Key interventions

- Measure oral temperature at least every 4 hours.
- Administer antipyretics, as prescribed.
- Observe for chills, diaphoresis, flushing, and hot, dry skin.
- Observe for seizures.
- Remove excess bed linens and clothing to promote heat loss.
- Offer fluids frequently.

- Keep room at temperature that is comfortable for the patient.

NURSING DIAGNOSIS

Pain related to inflammation

DESIRED PATIENT OUTCOME

The patient will experience relief from pain

Outcome measurement criteria

- ☐ Verbalization of decreased pain
- ☐ Vital signs within normal ranges
- ☐ Absence of nuchal rigidity and headache
- ☐ Absence of nausea and vomiting
- ☐ Relaxed facial expression and muscle tone

Key interventions

- Administer nonnarcotic analgesics, as prescribed, and document effectiveness. Inform patient of expected onset of analgesic action.
- Assess for signs and symptoms of pain, including changes in vital signs, facial grimaces, restlessness, shallow breathing, muscle tension, nausea, and vomiting.
- Apply ice pack to the patient's head to reduce pain.
- Explain principles of pain management to the patient and family, including meaning of *p.r.n.*
- Provide appropriate interventions to decrease anxiety associated with pain. For instance, listen to the patient's concerns and teach deep-breathing techniques.
- Avoid sudden, jarring movements, loud noises, and noxious odors, which may intensify pain.

- Close window blinds and keep lights dim to minimize photophobia.

NURSING DIAGNOSIS

High risk for fluid volume deficit related to fever

DESIRED PATIENT OUTCOME

The patient will maintain adequate hydration

Outcome measurement criteria

- ☐ Adequate skin turgor
- ☐ Adequate fluid balance
- ☐ Vital signs within normal ranges
- ☐ Urine specific gravity within normal range
- ☐ Serum electrolyte levels within normal ranges
- ☐ Absence of excessive thirst
- ☐ Maintenance of stable weight

Key interventions

- Monitor vital signs every 4 hours.
- Observe for signs and symptoms of dehydration, including poor skin turgor, dry skin, excessive thirst, and weight loss.
- Monitor urine specific gravity and serum electrolyte levels.
- Weigh the patient daily and record results.
- Determine the patient's fluid preferences and provide appropriate beverages frequently. Encourage the family to offer fluids during visits.
- Document fluid intake and output carefully.

NURSING DIAGNOSIS

Fear related to uncertainty regarding disease process

DESIRED PATIENT OUTCOME

The patient will demonstrate decreased fear

Outcome measurement criteria

- ☐ Verbalization of fears and concerns
- ☐ Participation in care and treatment within physiologic limitations
- ☐ Verbalization of understanding of disease process and realistic expectations for recovery
- ☐ Verbalization of ability to get adequate sleep

Key interventions

- Encourage the patient and family to discuss fears and concerns.
- Provide information about disease progression and signs and symptoms of recovery.
- Observe for signs of increasing fear or anxiety, and intervene promptly.
- Reassure the patient and family that symptoms usually are transient and recovery usually is complete.
- Explain all diagnostic tests and treatments. Stay with the patient during procedures.
- Explain purpose of antibiotic therapy and emphasize need to continue taking prescribed medication after discharge.
- Discuss importance of follow-up care during convalescence. Encourage the patient to allow ample time for recuperation before resuming normal schedule.

Multiple sclerosis

Progressive neurologic disease characterized by demyelination of nerve fibers of brain and spinal cord.

NURSING DIAGNOSIS

High risk for ineffective airway clearance related to fatigue and muscle weakness

DESIRED PATIENT OUTCOME

The patient will maintain a patent airway

Outcome measurement criteria

- ☐ Patent airway
- ☐ Decreased secretions
- ☐ Absence of adventitious lung sounds
- ☐ Absence of dyspnea and cyanosis
- ☐ Demonstration of effective coughing
- ☐ Demonstration of ability to expectorate secretions
- ☐ Absence of signs of aspiration

Key interventions

- Assess lung sounds and respiratory rate and effort every 4 hours. Document rhonchi, crackles, or wheezes.
- Suction airway, as needed.
- Keep head of bed elevated 45 degrees to promote breathing.
- Offer fluids to help liquefy secretions. Withhold dairy products, which increase mucus viscosity.

- Schedule rest periods between activities to conserve the patient's energy.
- Reposition the patient every 2 hours to help mobilize secretions.
- Teach the patient effective coughing and deep-breathing techniques. Observe return demonstrations.

NURSING DIAGNOSIS

Impaired physical mobility related to muscle weakness

DESIRED PATIENT OUTCOME

The patient will demonstrate optimal mobility

Outcome measurement criteria

- ☐ Demonstration of ability to move from bed to chair
- ☐ Demonstration of ability to ambulate within physiologic limitations
- ☐ Demonstration of correct use of assistive devices
- ☐ Participation in activities of daily living within limitations
- ☐ Demonstration of correct technique for range-of-motion (ROM) exercises
- ☐ Participation in physical therapy program
- ☐ Absence of complications of immobility, such as pneumonia, venous stasis, thrombus, and skin breakdown

Key interventions

- Assess the patient's functional ability on admission, and monitor for changes daily.
- During periods of bed rest, perform ROM exercises every 4 hours and reposition the patient every 2 hours.

- Provide assistance with progressive mobility as the patient's ability and strength permit.
- Schedule rest periods between activities to reduce fatigue.
- Monitor for complications of immobility.
- Use pressure relief mattress and other devices to help prevent skin breakdown.
- Apply antiembolism stockings, as ordered, to prevent venous stasis. Remove stockings for 1 hour each shift and then reapply.
- Encourage the patient and family to participate in prescribed exercise regimen.
- Emphasize need to monitor temperature of bath or shower water and to avoid heating pads.
- Instruct the patient to avoid activity after bathing or showering, when muscle strength is reduced.

NURSING DIAGNOSIS

Self-care deficit: bathing and/or toileting related to neuromuscular impairment secondary to demyelination

DESIRED PATIENT OUTCOME

The patient will perform self-care activities with minimal assistance

Outcome measurement criteria

- ☐ Verbalization of self-care needs
- ☐ Participation in self-care activities within physiologic limitations
- ☐ Verbalization of concerns and frustrations
- ☐ Demonstration of decreased need for assistance with self-care activities

☐ Demonstration of correct use of assistive devices

Key interventions

- Assess the patient's functional abilities and limitations on admission, and monitor for changes daily.
- Encourage the patient and family to discuss their concerns and frustrations. Reassure them that frustration is normal response to situation.
- Anticipate hygiene and toileting needs to decrease frustration.
- Offer bedpan, commode, or assistance to bathroom every 2 to 4 hours.
- Keep call button within the patient's reach at all times.
- Support efforts at independence. Encourage the patient to participate in daily care activities. Offer assistance as needed.
- Provide positive reinforcement for participation and progressive improvement in self-care activities.
- Provide assistive devices to promote independence. Teach the patient and family how to use these devices.
- Maintain safe environment.
- Provide privacy during bathing and dressing. Do not rush the patient through these activities.
- Teach the patient and family about home care.
- Encourage the family to bring clothing that the patient can put on and remove easily.
- Consult the occupational therapist for an evaluation of the patient's ability to perform self-care activities.

NURSING DIAGNOSIS

High risk for reflex incontinence related to neuromuscular impairment secondary to disease process

DESIRED PATIENT OUTCOME

The patient will establish and maintain a regular urine elimination pattern

Outcome measurement criteria

☐ Demonstration of ability to recognize need to void

☐ Communication of elimination needs to caregiver

☐ Participation in bladder retraining program

☐ Demonstration of bladder continence

☐ Absence of urine retention and urinary tract infection

Key interventions

- Discuss usual bladder habits with the patient to determine normal routines.
- Monitor fluid intake and output to help evaluate fluid balance.
- Advise the patient to drink at least 2,500 ml of fluid daily, unless contraindicated. Limit fluid intake after 7 p.m. to avoid nighttime incontinence.
- Anticipate toileting needs. Offer bedpan, commode, or assistance to bathroom every 2 hours.
- Stimulate urination by running tap water, providing glass of water, or stimulating skin on abdomen or thigh.
- Encourage the patient to wear protective pads under garments.
- Teach the patient and caregiver correct technique for intermittent bladder catheterization, if ordered and necessary. Observe return demonstration.
- Teach the patient and family about bladder routine that the patient should follow at home.

NURSING DIAGNOSIS

High risk for bowel incontinence related to neuromuscular impairment secondary to disease

DESIRED PATIENT OUTCOME

The patient will establish and maintain a regular bowel elimination pattern

Outcome measurement criteria

- ☐ Demonstration of ability to recognize the need to move bowels
- ☐ Verbalization of elimination needs to caregiver
- ☐ Demonstration of bowel continence
- ☐ Participation in bowel retraining program
- ☐ Absence of constipation or fecal impaction

Key interventions

- Discuss usual bowel habits with the patient to determine normal routines.
- Help the patient establish bowel routine, such as by offering warm beverage at breakfast, providing increased dietary fiber, and encouraging suppository use every other day.
- Anticipate toileting needs. Offer bedpan, commode, or assistance to bathroom every 2 hours.
- Teach the patient and family about bowel routine that the patient should follow at home.
- Monitor fluid intake and output.

NURSING DIAGNOSIS

Altered role performance related to perception of physical limitations

DESIRED PATIENT OUTCOME

The patient will demonstrate positive strategies for coping with role expectations

Outcome measurement criteria

- ☐ Verbalization of realistic role expectations
- ☐ Verbalization of strategies for coping with role changes
- ☐ Demonstration of application of positive coping skills
- ☐ Demonstration of acceptance of physical limitations
- ☐ Verbalization of personal strengths and capabilities
- ☐ Demonstration of successful redefinition of role

Key interventions

- Encourage the patient to discuss concerns and feelings.
- Provide environment that is conducive to open discussion and problem solving.
- Help the patient set realistic goals for role achievement.
- Provide feedback and reinforcement for positive behavior.
- Encourage the patient to continue to fulfill roles within physiologic limitations.
- Help the patient identify ways to adapt to illness by redefining role.
- Include the family in discussions, as appropriate.
- Teach the patient and family how to manage disease after discharge.
- Consult the social services department for assistance and counseling.

Parkinson's disease

Progressive, degenerative disease characterized by muscle rigidity, shuffling gait, resting tremors, and bradykinesia; associated with characteristic pathologic findings, such as degeneration within extrapyramidal brain nuclei and dopamine deficiency in corpus striatum.

NURSING DIAGNOSIS

Impaired physical mobility related to muscle weakness, rigidity, and tremors

DESIRED PATIENT OUTCOME

The patient will maintain optimal mobility

Outcome measurement criteria

- ☐ Demonstration of ambulation to highest level possible
- ☐ Demonstration of correct use of assistive devices
- ☐ Participation in activities of daily living to tolerance level
- ☐ Absence of complications of immobility, such as pneumonia, venous stasis, thrombus, and skin breakdown
- ☐ Demonstration of correct technique for range-of-motion (ROM) exercises
- ☐ Participation in physical therapy program

Key interventions

- Assess the patient's functional ability on admission, and monitor for changes daily.
- During periods of bed rest, perform ROM exercises every 4 hours and reposition the patient every 2 hours.

- Provide assistance with progressive mobility as the patient's ability and strength permit.
- Provide raised chair and toilet seat, and place head of bed or chair on blocks to help the patient sit and stand.
- Schedule rest periods between activities to reduce fatigue and muscle weakness.
- Advise the patient to avoid shuffling gait and to lift legs and stand erect when walking.
- Monitor for complications of immobility.
- Apply antiembolism stockings, as ordered, to help prevent venous stasis. Remove stockings for 1 hour each shift and then reapply.
- Encourage the patient and family to participate in prescribed exercise regimen.
- Consult the physical therapist regarding possible need for gait retraining program.

NURSING DIAGNOSIS

High risk for trauma related to unsteady gait and tremors

DESIRED PATIENT OUTCOME

The patient will remain free of injury

Outcome measurement criteria

- ☐ Absence of signs and symptoms of physical injury
- ☐ Verbalization of understanding of environmental hazards
- ☐ Demonstration of safe ambulation with assistance
- ☐ Consistent use of call button to request assistance
- ☐ Demonstration of correct use of assistive devices

Key interventions

- Assess the patient's abilities and limitations on admission, and monitor for changes daily.
- Determine the patient's degree of physical risk, based on established criteria.
- Implement safety protocol according to hospital policy.
- Assess environment for such hazards as dim lights, spills, and slippery floors.
- Provide adequate lighting to illuminate all areas used by the patient and to eliminate shadows.
- Keep call button within the patient's reach at all times, and encourage its use as needed.
- Teach the patient and family how to use assistive devices correctly. Observe return demonstration.
- Schedule rest periods to decrease fatigue and risk of injury.
- Assist the patient at meals, as necessary. Allow hot beverages to cool slightly before giving them to the patient.
- Provide shower seat and hand rails in bathroom. Do not leave the patient unattended in bathroom.
- Ask the family to bring nonskid shoes or slippers for the patient.
- Instruct the family to evaluate home for environmental hazards and to remove or modify hazards before the patient is discharged.

NURSING DIAGNOSIS

Body image disturbance related to diminishing functional abilities

DESIRED PATIENT OUTCOME

The patient will verbalize acceptance of bodily changes

Outcome measurement criteria

- ☐ Verbalization of concerns and feelings
- ☐ Verbalization of realistic expectations about diminishing functional abilities
- ☐ Participation in daily activities to tolerance level
- ☐ Verbalization of physical, emotional, intellectual, and spiritual strengths
- ☐ Demonstration of ability to compensate for functional limitations

Key interventions

- Encourage the patient to discuss concerns and feelings about diminishing functional abilities.
- Assist the patient in identifying physical, emotional, intellectual, and spiritual strengths.
- Suggest use of assistive devices to help compensate for functional limitations.
- Offer physical assistance as needed.
- Encourage participation in self-care activities, and offer positive reinforcement for the patient's efforts.
- Assist the family in recognizing effects of the patient's limitations.
- Consult with the social services department regarding the patient's counseling needs.

NURSING DIAGNOSIS

High risk for caregiver role strain related to effects of neuromuscular deficits, cognitive deficits, or both

DESIRED PATIENT OUTCOME

The caregiver will develop positive strategies for dealing with role strain

Outcome measurement criteria

- ☐ Verbalization of current stressors
- ☐ Verbalization of effects of role strain on daily life
- ☐ Verbalization of feelings about competing roles
- ☐ Demonstration of positive coping strategies for dealing with role strain
- ☐ Verbalization of need for respite help and recreation
- ☐ Demonstration of acceptance of help from family, friends, and outside agencies in managing responsibilities

Key interventions

- Encourage the caregiver to discuss feelings and concerns. Use open, nonjudgmental approach to promote trusting relationship.
- Help the caregiver identify and acknowledge specific stressors that increase role strain.
- Discuss coping skills the caregiver has used successfully in past. Assist in adapting these skills to present situation.
- Discuss diversional activities, and explore ways to incorporate these into the caregiver's daily routine.
- Identify areas of knowledge deficit. Provide appropriate information to help reduce role strain.
- Assist in identifying support systems, such as family members, friends, religious institution, and clergy.
- Obtain information from the social services department regarding available community resources and long-term care placement options, if necessary.

Seizure disorder

Disorder characterized by disturbance of brain's electrical activity; may be accompanied by alterations in behavior and level of consciousness (LOC), impaired autonomic function, and sudden, violent muscle contractions.

NURSING DIAGNOSIS

High risk for trauma related to altered LOC and impaired autonomic function

DESIRED PATIENT OUTCOME

The patient will remain free of injury

Outcome measurement criteria

☐ Absence of signs and symptoms of injury

☐ Alertness and orientation to person, place, and time

☐ Absence of seizures

Key interventions

- Implement seizure precautions, such as padding side rails, keeping bed in low position, and keeping oral airway and suction equipment at bedside.
- Monitor neurologic status.
- Keep call button within the patient's reach at all times.
- If seizure occurs, turn the patient onto side to keep airway open. Do not attempt to place anything in mouth during seizure. Provide privacy, and stay with the patient.
- If seizure occurs when the patient is out of bed, ease the patient onto floor and support and protect the patient's head.

- Observe and document type and duration of seizure, body parts involved, and neurologic status before and after seizure.
- After seizure ends, monitor vital signs and reorient the patient. Provide oral hygiene and suctioning as needed.
- Reassure the patient and family that patient safety will be maintained if seizures occur.

NURSING DIAGNOSIS

Anxiety related to change in health status secondary to seizure disorder

DESIRED PATIENT OUTCOME

The patient will exhibit decreased anxiety

Outcome measurement criteria

- ☐ Verbalization of concerns and fears
- ☐ Absence or decrease in anxiety
- ☐ Vital signs within normal ranges
- ☐ Relaxed facial expression and muscle tone
- ☐ Verbalization of understanding of disorder, treatment, and preventive measures

Key interventions

- Encourage the patient to discuss concerns and fears about seizure disorder.
- Provide accurate information and dispel myths about seizure disorder. Encourage the patient and family to ask questions.
- Discuss the patient's perception of how seizures affect life-style.
- Encourage the patient to maintain positive attitude toward disorder and its management.

- Teach the family safety precautions to take during seizures.
- Advise the patient to explain seizure-related safety precautions to friends and coworkers.
- Encourage the patient to continue normal activities and daily routines.
- Caution the patient to avoid excessive stress or emotional upset because this may precipitate seizures.
- Discuss prescribed medications and emphasize importance of complying with prescribed administration schedule.
- Stress need for follow-up care, including periodic blood tests to check for drug toxicity.
- Caution the patient not to take over-the-counter medications unless the primary health care practitioner approves.
- Provide application for Medic-Alert identification.

NURSING DIAGNOSIS

Social isolation related to embarrassment associated with changes in appearance and behavior during seizures

DESIRED PATIENT OUTCOME

The patient will establish a plan for increasing social activity

Outcome measurement criteria

☐ Verbalization of feelings about social isolation

☐ Open communication with caregivers

☐ Verbalization of desire to participate in family or social activities after discharge and to return to work or school

☐ Verbalization of understanding of seizure disorder, its treatment, and preventive measures

- ☐ Verbalization of decreased feelings of isolation
- ☐ Demonstration of increased social activity during hospital stay

Key interventions

- Encourage the patient to express concerns and feelings about seizure disorder and perceived need for isolation.
- Discuss specific situations in which the patient feels unable to participate, such as work, social activities, and sports. Help the patient find ways to maintain participation.
- Provide accurate information about seizure disorder, its treatment, and preventive measures. Clarify misconceptions.
- Encourage and provide positive reinforcement for participation in self-care and diversional activities.
- Provide ample time for visits with family and friends.
- Encourage social interaction with staff and other patients, as appropriate.
- Refer the patient to local classes and support groups for continuing interaction and support.

Spinal cord injury

Injury to spinal cord, which may cause loss of motor and sensory function at and below injury level.

NURSING DIAGNOSIS

High risk for impaired skin integrity related to prolonged immobility

DESIRED PATIENT OUTCOME

The patient will remain free of skin breakdown

Outcome measurement criteria

- ☐ Warm, dry skin
- ☐ Strong peripheral pulses
- ☐ Adequate skin turgor
- ☐ Normal skin color
- ☐ Adequate fluid intake and output
- ☐ Absence of redness, blistering, and edema (signs of impending or actual skin breakdown)
- ☐ Serum albumin and protein values within normal ranges

Key interventions

- Assess skin integrity at least every 4 hours. Observe for redness, blistering, and edema, especially over bony prominences.
- Monitor skin turgor for evidence of dehydration.
- Palpate peripheral pulses.
- Assess skin temperature and capillary refill time.

- Document fluid intake and output to help assess fluid balance.
- Encourage activity within physiologic limitations.
- Turn and reposition the patient with pillows every 2 hours.
- Maintain proper body alignment using pillows, towel rolls, splints, and high-top sneakers.
- Keep skin clean and dry. Lubricate with lotion or oil.
- Use draw sheets to move the patient in bed.
- Use air mattress, heel and elbow pads, and other appropriate preventive devices.
- Perform passive or active range-of-motion exercises on affected arms and legs.
- Monitor serum albumin and protein values to help assess nutritional status.
- Teach the patient and family preventive skin care techniques. Observe return demonstration before discharge.

NURSING DIAGNOSIS

Body image disturbance related to diminished motor and sensory function

DESIRED PATIENT OUTCOME

The patient will verbalize acceptance of bodily changes

Outcome measurement criteria

- ☐ Verbalization of concerns and feelings
- ☐ Verbalization of realistic expectations regarding body image changes
- ☐ Participation in daily activities to tolerance level

- ☐ Verbalization of physical, emotional, intellectual, and spiritual strengths
- ☐ Demonstration of ability to compensate for limited functional abilities

Key interventions

- Encourage the patient to discuss concerns and feelings, including anger and grief.
- Recognize that the patient's anger is not directed at the nurse personally.
- Identify manipulative or disruptive behavior, and set limits on such behavior.
- Explain the patient's behavior to the family to foster understanding and patience.
- Help the patient identify physical, emotional, intellectual, and spiritual strengths.
- Suggest use of assistive devices to help compensate for certain limitations.
- Offer physical assistance as needed.
- Encourage and offer positive reinforcement for participation in self-care activities.
- Help the family recognize personal, social, financial, and medical implications of the patient's condition.
- Consult the social services department regarding counseling needs.

NURSING DIAGNOSIS

Urinary retention related to motor and sensory deficits secondary to spinal cord injury

DESIRED PATIENT OUTCOME

The patient will demonstrate adequate bladder emptying

Outcome measurement criteria

- ☐ Verbalization of feeling of comfort
- ☐ Absence of bladder distention
- ☐ Adequate fluid balance
- ☐ Urinalysis results within normal range
- ☐ Absence of signs and symptoms of urinary tract infection

Key interventions

- Discuss normal voiding patterns with the patient and monitor current patterns to establish baseline.
- Monitor fluid intake and output.
- Encourage fluid intake of 2,500 ml/day, unless contraindicated. Limit fluids after 7 p.m. to avoid nocturnal incontinence or need for self-catheterization at night.
- Palpate bladder for distention.
- Perform bladder credé every 2 to 3 hours to promote voiding.
- Monitor urinalysis results for evidence of infection.
- Perform intermittent catheterization, as ordered. Teach the patient or family correct catheterization technique. Observe return demonstration.
- Teach the patient and family to observe for signs and symptoms of bladder fullness, including restlessness, diaphoresis, and chills.

NURSING DIAGNOSIS

Bowel incontinence related to motor and sensory deficits secondary to spinal cord injury

DESIRED PATIENT OUTCOME

The patient will maintain adequate bowel control

Outcome measurement criteria

- ☐ Participation in bowel retraining program
- ☐ Demonstration of adequate bowel control
- ☐ Verbalization of understanding of bowel retraining program
- ☐ Verbalization of signs and symptoms of bowel fullness
- ☐ Absence of fecal impaction

Key interventions

- Determine the patient's previous bowel habits.
- Discuss bowel retraining program with the patient and family.
- Establish goals of bowel training program with the patient.
- Help the patient establish bowel routine, such as by serving warm beverage at breakfast, providing dietary bran, and administering suppositories every other day.
- Encourage the patient to drink at least 2,500 ml/day of fluid, unless contraindicated.
- Advise the patient to consume adequate dietary fiber and to avoid gas-forming foods.
- Anticipate toileting needs. Offer bedpan or commode every 2 hours.
- Teach the patient how to recognize signs and symptoms of full bowel, including perspiration, goose bumps, and sense of fullness.
- Teach the patient to stimulate defecation by massaging abdomen or applying pressure to inner thigh.

NURSING DIAGNOSIS

High risk for dysreflexia related to noxious stimuli

DESIRED PATIENT OUTCOME

The patient will remain free of complications associated with dysreflexia

Outcome measurement criteria

- ☐ Return of blood pressure and heart rate to within normal ranges
- ☐ Absence of bladder or bowel distention
- ☐ Absence of diaphoresis, chilling, headache, nasal congestion, and nausea
- ☐ Verbalization of factors that precipitate dysreflexia
- ☐ Communication of signs and symptoms of dysreflexia to staff

Key interventions

- Assess for signs and symptoms of dysreflexia, including sudden rise in blood pressure, change in heart rate, headache, diaphoresis, and blotchy skin.
- Determine precipitating factor for dysreflexia episode, and take measures to eliminate it.
- Check catheter tubing for kinks and attempt to stimulate voiding if the patient's bladder is distended.
- Check carefully for fecal impaction. Remove impaction as needed, using anesthetic lubricant to decrease stimulation.
- Monitor vital signs frequently.
- Elevate head of bed and lower the patient's legs to counteract hypertension.

- Assess environment for factors that may precipitate dysreflexia, such as drafts or objects that put pressure on skin.
- Teach the patient and family how to prevent dysreflexia.

NURSING DIAGNOSIS

Altered sexuality patterns related to motor and sensory deficits secondary to spinal cord injury

DESIRED PATIENT OUTCOME

The patient will communicate concerns about sexuality

Outcome measurement criteria

- ☐ Verbalization of concerns about sexuality
- ☐ Verbalization of realistic expectations about sexuality
- ☐ Demonstration of effective communication about sexuality between the patient and significant other, if applicable
- ☐ Verbalization of desire to use counseling services to address sexuality issues

Key interventions

- Provide uninterrupted time with the patient to discuss sexuality issues.
- Encourage discussion by letting the patient know that concerns about sexuality after spinal cord injury are normal. For example, use such phrases as "Many patients experience..." or "Other patients express concern that ...," followed by "How do you feel about that?"
- Use nonjudgmental approach and maintain atmosphere conducive to open discussion.

- Provide accurate information and clarify misconceptions about effects of spinal cord injury on sexuality.
- Refer the patient and significant other to an appropriate counselor for follow-up after discharge.

Diabetes mellitus

Chronic disorder of carbohydrate, protein, and fat metabolism caused by deficiency or complete lack of insulin.

NURSING DIAGNOSIS

Altered nutrition: more than body requirements related to excessive food intake, established eating habits, and lack of information about proper nutrition

DESIRED PATIENT OUTCOME

The patient will maintain appropriate nutritional intake

Outcome measurement criteria

- ☐ Consumption of prescribed types and amounts of food
- ☐ Gradual weight reduction (1 to 2 lb [0.45 to 0.9 kg] per week)
- ☐ Control of blood glucose level
- ☐ Adherence to dietary restrictions
- ☐ Selection of proper food portions
- ☐ Verbalization of how food intake and exercise affect blood glucose level

Key interventions

- Evaluate normal eating habits. Encourage the patient to keep food diary to monitor nutritional intake.
- Monitor fingerstick blood glucose levels, as ordered.
- Weigh the patient daily.
- Monitor and document daily food intake.

- Explain how food intake and exercise affect blood glucose level.
- Teach the patient and family how to use food exchange system or count carbohydrates to meet dietary requirements.
- Emphasize importance of controlling food portions to maintain or lose weight and to control blood glucose level.
- Stress that the patient must eat meals and snacks on regular schedule to avoid blood glucose extremes.
- Observe the patient's ability to select correct types and amounts of food from hospital menu. Help the patient make appropriate choices, as needed.
- Provide sample meal plans and educational materials for use as at-home references.
- Consult the dietitian for further nutritional assessment and patient education.

NURSING DIAGNOSIS

High risk for fluid volume deficit related to excessive urine output secondary to elevated blood glucose level

DESIRED PATIENT OUTCOME

The patient will maintain adequate fluid balance

Outcome measurement criteria

- ☐ Balanced fluid intake and output
- ☐ Heart rate and blood pressure within normal ranges
- ☐ Adequate skin turgor
- ☐ Adequate hydration of mucous membranes
- ☐ Hematocrit value within normal range
- ☐ Urine specific gravity within normal range

☐ Demonstration of adequate fluid intake

Key interventions

- Monitor and document fluid intake and output every shift.
- Initiate I.V. fluid replacement, if necessary and prescribed.
- Observe for signs of dehydration, such as poor skin turgor, dry mucous membranes, tachycardia, and decreased blood pressure.
- Monitor urine specific gravity and hematocrit values to help assess fluid status.
- Encourage the patient to drink noncaloric fluids during hyperglycemic episodes to replace fluid loss.

NURSING DIAGNOSIS

High risk for impaired skin integrity related to altered circulation and sensory and perceptual changes

DESIRED PATIENT OUTCOME

The patient will maintain adequate skin integrity

Outcome measurement criteria

☐ Presence of pedal pulses

☐ Capillary refill less than 3 seconds

☐ Normal skin color and temperature

☐ Absence of redness, blisters, inflammation, and skin breaks

☐ Absence of signs and symptoms of infection

☐ Demonstration of proper foot care

☐ Verbalization of importance of seeking medical attention at first sign of skin breakdown

☐ Identification of signs and symptoms of infection

Key interventions

- Assess skin integrity, pedal pulses, capillary refill time, and skin color and temperature in both legs during each shift while the patient is awake.
- Observe legs for cuts, cracks, blisters, redness, and other signs of skin infection or breakdown. Pay special attention to areas between toes.
- Inspect feet for calluses, corns, and ingrown toenails. Consult a podiatrist, as needed.
- Keep the patient's feet clean and dry. Bathe feet daily. Apply lubricating cream if skin is dry and cracked. Apply powder if feet become moist with perspiration.
- Teach the patient to inspect feet daily, using a mirror to view soles.
- Discourage self-treatment of corns, calluses, and ingrown toenails. Refer the patient to a podiatrist.
- Caution the patient never to wear tight-fitting shoes or walk barefoot.
- Advise the patient to avoid practices that may impede leg circulation, such as smoking, crossing legs, wearing garters or tight-fitting leg garments, and exposing legs to extreme cold.
- Teach the patient how to perform leg exercises that promote circulation. Consult the physical therapist to develop exercise plan and provide patient teaching. Reinforce teaching daily.
- Advise the patient to keep bath water at 85° to 90° F (about 30° to 32° C) and to test water with thermometer before immersing feet to avoid burns.
- Discourage use of heating pads and hot water bottles. Caution the patient not to warm feet against fireplaces or radiators.

- Encourage the patient to report signs and symptoms of infection and nonhealing wounds to the primary health care practitioner.

NURSING DIAGNOSIS

Ineffective management of therapeutic regimen related to lack of information and complexity of required lifestyle changes

DESIRED PATIENT OUTCOME

The patient will exhibit the skills and understanding required to manage diabetes effectively

Outcome measurement criteria

- ☐ Verbalization of concerns and fears about diabetes and its management
- ☐ Verbalization of need for lifestyle changes
- ☐ Adherence to dietary requirements
- ☐ Participation in diabetes management plan
- ☐ Demonstration of correct technique for preparing and administering insulin, if prescribed
- ☐ Adherence to medication regimen
- ☐ Demonstration of correct blood glucose monitoring technique
- ☐ Discussion of signs and symptoms of hypoglycemia and its treatment
- ☐ Verbalization of how food intake, exercise, and medication affect blood glucose level
- ☐ Description of diabetes management during periods of illness
- ☐ Identification of appropriate community resources

Key interventions

- Assess the patient's knowledge of diabetes management. Identify barriers to learning, such as language and communication deficits, illiteracy, cognitive or visual impairment, emotional upset, and cultural and socio-economic factors.
- Explain diabetes pathophysiology in simple terms. Give the patient time to ask questions and discuss concerns.
- Stress need for routine blood glucose monitoring to determine how food intake, exercise, and medication affect blood glucose level.
- Teach the patient how to measure blood glucose level, using a glucose monitor. Observe several return demonstrations to ensure mastery.
- Teach the patient how to clean and maintain glucose monitor. Provide manufacturer's toll-free customer service number in case problems occur after discharge.
- Provide log book in which the patient can document blood glucose levels, medications administered, and food intake.
- Discuss effects of exercise on blood glucose level. Encourage the patient to get regular exercise at least three times weekly.
- Explain medication regimen, including type, name, purpose, dosage, and common adverse effects of prescribed insulin.
- Teach correct technique for insulin preparation and injection. Observe several return demonstrations to ensure mastery.
- Instruct the patient to administer insulin at room temperature to aid absorption. Explain that bottle in use may be kept at room temperature for 1 month, but extra bottles should be refrigerated.
- Emphasize importance of rotating insulin injection sites.

- Instruct the patient to stay alert for signs and symptoms of hypoglycemia, such as nervousness, weakness, perspiration, confusion, headache, irritability, and trembling. Be aware that these classic signs and symptoms may not occur if the patient is taking human insulin. Also, hypoglycemia may mimic cerebrovascular accident in an elderly patient. Encourage the patient to report unusual signs and symptoms to the primary health care practitioner.
- Stress need for prompt treatment of hypoglycemia. Instruct the patient to ingest quickly absorbed glucose source, such as half cup of fruit juice or cola, four sugar cubes, or two graham crackers, to raise blood glucose level. Encourage the patient to keep glucose tablets on hand.
- Advise the patient to note hypoglycemic episodes in daily log.
- Reinforce the dietitian's instructions. Provide sample meal plans and food exchange lists for the patient and family to use as references.
- Have the patient select appropriate foods from sample menus of fast-food and other restaurants to assess comprehension of teaching.
- Discuss sick-day guidelines, including how to manage diabetes on days when illness alters the patient's usual diet. Instruct the patient to monitor blood glucose and urine ketone levels more frequently, increase intake of nondietetic fluids, and spread 50% of normal carbohydrate allowance over 24-hour period. Advise the patient to contact the primary health care practitioner early in course of illness to discuss possible adjustment of insulin dosage and other measures.
- Discuss potential diabetes complications, such as retinopathy, peripheral neuropathy, and kidney disease.
- Encourage the patient to have annual eye examinations and report visual changes immediately.

- Provide list of community resources, including diabetes support groups, weight management groups, smoking cessation classes, and stress management programs.
- Refer the patient and family to outpatient diabetes management program for follow-up care.

Hyperthyroidism

Disorder of excessive thyroid function and excess thyroid hormone secretion characterized by such signs and symptoms as goiter, tachycardia, palpitations, hypertension, poor concentration, anxiety, irritability, increased appetite, heat intolerance, excessive sweating, weight loss, tremors, and muscle weakness.

NURSING DIAGNOSIS

High risk for altered body temperature related to increased metabolism and thyroid hormone secretion secondary to thyroid storm (hyperthyroid crisis)

DESIRED PATIENT OUTCOME

The patient will maintain a normal body temperature

Outcome measurement criteria

- ☐ Oral temperature at or below 99.0° F (37.2° C)
- ☐ Heart rate within normal range
- ☐ Serum thyroid hormone levels within normal ranges
- ☐ Absence of respiratory distress
- ☐ Absence of restlessness, apprehension, and irritability
- ☐ Orientation to person, place, and time

Key interventions

- Measure oral temperature at least every 4 hours. Be aware that temperature may rise spontaneously to 106.0° F (41.1° C).
- Monitor for tachycardia and respiratory distress caused by increased metabolic rate.

- Observe for signs and symptoms of thyroid storm, such as irritability, restlessness, apprehension, and heat intolerance.
- Observe for changes in level of consciousness. Be aware that delirium and coma may occur if thyroid storm goes untreated.
- Notify the physician immediately of elevated temperature or other signs and symptoms of thyroid storm.
- Monitor serum thyroid hormone levels daily and report significant changes to the physician.
- Administer I.V. fluid therapy, as prescribed, to improve hydration.
- Keep the patient's room at comfortable temperature.
- Advise the patient to wear lightweight clothing and use lightweight bed sheets and blankets.

NURSING DIAGNOSIS

Altered nutrition: less than body requirements related to increased metabolic demand

DESIRED PATIENT OUTCOME

The patient will maintain adequate nutritional intake

Outcome measurement criteria

☐ Adherence to prescribed diet

☐ Maintenance of stable weight

☐ Hemoglobin and serum albumin levels within normal ranges

Key interventions

- Weigh the patient daily.
- Monitor daily food intake.

- Provide meals high in calories, protein, and carbohydrates.
- Encourage the patient to eat six small meals daily or to snack between meals.
- Discourage consumption of caffeinated foods and beverages because they have a stimulant effect.
- Monitor hemoglobin and serum albumin levels. Report significant changes to the physician.
- Consult the dietitian for additional nutritional assessment and patient education.

NURSING DIAGNOSIS

Ineffective individual coping related to emotional lability

DESIRED PATIENT OUTCOME

The patient will exhibit appropriate coping mechanisms to minimize emotional lability

Outcome measurement criteria

- ☐ Verbalization and demonstration of decreased nervousness
- ☐ Absence of manic behavior
- ☐ Demonstration of improved fine motor coordination
- ☐ Demonstration of improved concentration
- ☐ Demonstration of decreased irritability
- ☐ Use of appropriate coping mechanisms

Key interventions

- Assess for nervousness, anxiety, and irritability.
- Observe the patient's ability to concentrate on specific tasks and perform activities that require fine motor coordination.

- Explain causes of behavioral changes to the patient and family to foster understanding and patience.
- Discourage ingestion of stimulants, such as coffee, tea, and alcohol.
- Maintain calm, relaxed environment.
- Discuss coping strategies the patient has used in past to deal with difficult situations or emotional lability. Encourage the patient to adapt these strategies to current situation.
- Provide written information and videotapes, if available, on stress management.
- Teach relaxation techniques, such as deep breathing, meditation, and guided imagery. Observe return demonstrations. Encourage use of these techniques during periods of stress or nervousness.
- Consult the social services department for additional counseling or referral.

NURSING DIAGNOSIS

High risk for injury related to inadequate protective mechanism of eyes

DESIRED PATIENT OUTCOME

The patient will remain free from corneal and conjunctival injury

Outcome measurement criteria

- ☐ Adequate conjunctival lubrication
- ☐ Absence of conjunctival redness, irritation, and pain
- ☐ Absence of vision changes
- ☐ Demonstration of correct technique for administering lubricating eye drops, ointment, or gel and applying eye patch

- ☐ Verbalization of importance of protecting eyes from sun, wind, and dust

Key interventions

- Assess the patient's ability to close eyes.
- Observe conjunctivae for redness, irritation, and dryness.
- Assess for eye pain.
- Administer lubricating eye drops or ointment frequently.
- Reassess the patient's need for lubricated eye patch or gel for increased protection.
- Teach the patient how to administer lubricating eye drops or ointment. Observe return demonstration.
- Instruct the patient to report vision changes immediately.
- Encourage the patient to wear dark glasses to protect eyes from sun, wind, and dust.

NURSING DIAGNOSIS

High risk for ineffective management of therapeutic regimen related to lack of information about follow-up care

DESIRED PATIENT OUTCOME

The patient will develop a plan to integrate the therapeutic regimen into daily life

Outcome measurement criteria

- ☐ Discussion of disease and its causes
- ☐ Identification of signs and symptoms to report
- ☐ Verbalization of medication regimen

- ☐ Adherence to medication regimen
- ☐ Verbalization of nutritional needs
- ☐ Verbalization of need for follow-up thyroid studies
- ☐ Description of thyroid surgery, if required

Key interventions

- Teach the patient and family about hyperthyroidism. Encourage them to express concerns and ask questions.
- Explain that medications used to treat hyperthyroidism may cause hypothyroidism. Instruct the patient to report signs and symptoms of hypothyroidism, such as weight gain, lethargy, dry skin, cold intolerance, constipation, and changes in hair texture.
- Review names, purposes, dosages, and common adverse effects of prescribed drugs.
- Demonstrate correct technique for administering eye drops. Observe return demonstration.
- Discuss the patient's nutritional needs. Reinforce importance of consuming diet high in calories, protein, and carbohydrates.
- Emphasize importance of follow-up thyroid studies to evaluate thyroid hormone levels and determine need for adjusting drug dosages.
- Discuss purpose and nature of thyroid surgery, if required.

Hypothyroidism

Disorder of deficient thyroid function and deficient thyroid hormone secretion characterized by such signs and symptoms as decreased basal metabolic rate, weight gain, fatigue, dry skin, changes in hair texture, constipation, cold intolerance, and menstrual disturbances.

NURSING DIAGNOSIS

High risk for decreased cardiac output related to reduced metabolic rate

DESIRED PATIENT OUTCOME

The patient will maintain adequate cardiac output

Outcome measurement criteria

☐ Heart rate and blood pressure within normal ranges

☐ Normal sinus cardiac rhythm

☐ Normal skin color and temperature

☐ Normal capillary refill time

☐ Adequate urine output

☐ Normal peripheral pulses

☐ Alertness and orientation to person, place, and time

Key interventions

- Monitor vital signs every 4 hours.
- Observe for changes in heart rhythm by auscultating heart or assessing electrocardiogram.
- Palpate peripheral pulses.
- Observe skin color and temperature.

- Monitor daily fluid intake and output.
- Weigh the patient daily.
- Observe for changes in level of consciousness.
- Administer lower dosages of sedatives and narcotics, as prescribed, because decreased metabolic rate potentiates effects of these drugs.

NURSING DIAGNOSIS

Activity intolerance related to fatigue

DESIRED PATIENT OUTCOME

The patient will gradually increase participation in self-care activities

Outcome measurement criteria

- ☐ Decrease in complaints of fatigue
- ☐ Increased participation in self-care activities, as tolerated
- ☐ Appropriate pacing of activities with rest periods
- ☐ Demonstration of ability to ambulate without dyspnea
- ☐ Demonstration of decreased need for rest

Key interventions

- Assess the patient's ability to participate in activities of daily living.
- Observe for complaints of fatigue, lethargy, and weakness.
- Assist with self-care activities, as needed.
- Provide positive reinforcement for increasing participation in activities.
- Schedule uninterrupted rest between care activities and procedures and tests to conserve the patient's energy.

- Use blankets, heavy robe, and socks to prevent hypothermia and conserve the patient's energy.

NURSING DIAGNOSIS

Constipation related to decreased metabolic rate

DESIRED PATIENT OUTCOME

The patient will regain normal bowel function

Outcome measurement criteria

- ☐ Resumption of normal bowel habits
- ☐ Presence of bowel sounds
- ☐ Absence of constipation and fecal impaction
- ☐ Soft, nontender abdomen
- ☐ Identification of high-fiber foods
- ☐ Consumption of adequate dietary fiber
- ☐ Adequate fluid intake
- ☐ Adherence to bowel retraining program, if applicable

Key interventions

- Evaluate the patient's normal bowel habits.
- Assess for bowel sounds and abdominal tightness and tenderness during each shift.
- Monitor fluid intake and output daily.
- Note complaints of constipation.
- Observe for fecal impaction, as necessary.
- Provide low-calorie, high-fiber, high-protein meals.
- Offer preferred fluids frequently.
- Establish daily bowel routine, including hot beverage and bran in morning, high-fiber foods throughout day, and suppositories every other day, as needed.

- Discuss role of fluid and dietary fiber in maintaining normal bowel activity.

NURSING DIAGNOSIS

Knowledge deficit regarding disorder, medication regimen, and follow-up care

DESIRED PATIENT OUTCOME

The patient will express an understanding of the disorder, medication regimen, and required follow-up care

Outcome measurement criteria

- ☐ Description of disorder
- ☐ Discussion of prescribed medication regimen
- ☐ Adherence to medication regimen
- ☐ Identification of dietary recommendations
- ☐ Identification of signs and symptoms of hypothyroidism and hyperthyroidism
- ☐ Verbalization of need for lifelong treatment
- ☐ Verbalization of need for follow-up thyroid studies

Key interventions

- Teach the patient and family about hypothyroidism.
- Discuss thyroid replacement therapy and need for periodic dosage adjustment.
- Review dietary guidelines. Provide written information about high-protein, high-fiber, low-calorie foods.
- Explain that medications used to treat hypothyroidism may cause hyperthyroidism. Instruct the patient to report signs and symptoms of hyperthyroidism, such as increased heart rate and blood pressure, anxiety, poor concentration, irritability, weight loss, increased appetite, and heat intolerance.

- Emphasize need for lifelong treatment to ensure necessary thyroid hormones to sustain life.
- Stress importance of periodic evaluation by the primary health care practitioner to evaluate effectiveness of treatment.

Thyroidectomy

Partial or complete removal of thyroid gland.

NURSING DIAGNOSIS

Fear related to impending surgery and postoperative recovery

DESIRED PATIENT OUTCOME

The patient will express decreased fear about surgery and its outcome

Outcome measurement criteria

- ☐ Verbalization of concerns and fears
- ☐ Discussion of surgery and postoperative care
- ☐ Relaxed facial expression and body posture
- ☐ Use of relaxation techniques to control fear
- ☐ Verbalization of decreased fear

Key interventions

- Assess the patient for anxiety and fear.
- Encourage the patient to express concerns and fears.
- Listen for verbal cues indicating increased or decreased fear.
- Explain all preoperative and postoperative care.
- Teach relaxation techniques, such as deep breathing, meditation, and guided imagery.
- Maintain environment that is conducive to relaxation.

NURSING DIAGNOSIS

High risk for ineffective airway clearance related to inflammation and edema secondary to surgical incision

DESIRED PATIENT OUTCOME

The patient will maintain a patent airway

Outcome measurement criteria

- ☐ Absence of obstructed airway
- ☐ Absence of apprehension, restlessness, and cyanosis
- ☐ Pulse oximetry values within normal ranges
- ☐ Decrease in edema
- ☐ Demonstration of ability to expectorate secretions
- ☐ Verbalization of ability to breathe comfortably

Key interventions

- Assess respiratory status according to postoperative protocol. Observe rate, depth, and character of respirations.
- Assess surgical incision for increasing edema. Note tightness of dressing and complaints of difficulty swallowing.
- Observe for apprehension, restlessness, and cyanosis, which signal impaired air exchange or airway obstruction.
- Monitor pulse oximetry values, as ordered, and report significant changes to the physician.
- Keep bed in semi-Fowler's position to promote comfortable breathing.
- Keep suction equipment and tracheostomy kit at bedside in case of tracheal obstruction.

NURSING DIAGNOSIS

High risk for fluid volume deficit related to potential postoperative hemorrhage

DESIRED PATIENT OUTCOME

The patient will maintain adequate fluid balance

Outcome measurement criteria

- ☐ Balanced fluid intake and output
- ☐ Vital signs within normal ranges
- ☐ Normal skin color and temperature
- ☐ Normal level of consciousness
- ☐ Hemoglobin and hematocrit values within normal ranges
- ☐ Absence of signs and symptoms of hemorrhage

Key interventions

- Measure vital signs frequently during immediate postoperative period. Observe for signs and symptoms of hemorrhage, such as decreased heart rate, reduced blood pressure, and cool, clammy skin.
- Assess surgical dressing at least every hour for excessive bleeding, especially at sides of neck and back of head.
- Monitor level of consciousness.
- Assess hemoglobin and hematocrit values, and report significant changes to the physician.

NURSING DIAGNOSIS

Pain related to inflammation secondary to surgical tissue trauma

DESIRED PATIENT OUTCOME

The patient will experience relief from pain

Outcome measurement criteria

- ☐ Verbalization of adequate pain relief
- ☐ Vital signs within normal ranges
- ☐ Relaxed facial expression and muscle tone
- ☐ Verbalization of ability to obtain adequate rest
- ☐ Demonstration of ability to use comfort measures

Key interventions

- Assess for evidence of pain, such as increased blood pressure, tachycardia, facial grimacing, shallow breathing, irritability, and restlessness.
- Explain principles of pain management, including meaning of *p.r.n.*
- Encourage the patient to request medication before pain becomes severe.
- Teach the patient how to use patient-controlled analgesia pump, if applicable.
- Monitor effectiveness of pain medication.
- Place the patient in semi-Fowler's position to promote comfort and breathing.
- Observe for edema around surgical incision.
- Logroll the patient's head and chest during repositioning to avoid strain on suture line.
- Teach the patient how to use rolled towel to support head and neck during movement.

NURSING DIAGNOSIS

Impaired verbal communication related to location of surgical incision

DESIRED PATIENT OUTCOME

The patient will maintain effective communication

Outcome measurement criteria

- ☐ Minimal changes in vocal tone or pitch
- ☐ Effective use of alternative communication method, if needed
- ☐ Expression of satisfaction with chosen communication method
- ☐ Consistent communication of needs to staff

Key interventions

- Discuss communication impairment with the patient and family.
- Reassure the patient that acceptable communication method will be established immediately.
- Provide selection of communication methods, such as paper and pen, Magic Slate, picture board, poster with common questions, and use of gestures.
- Monitor vocal pitch and tone every 1 to 2 hours to detect signs of vocal cord damage.
- Discourage the patient from talking to prevent vocal cord edema. Ask visitors to limit conversation that requires verbal response from the patient.
- Reassure the patient that hoarseness caused by edema will subside within several days.

Acute renal failure

Sudden, severe impairment or loss of renal function associated with increase in serum urea and creatinine levels.

NURSING DIAGNOSIS

Fluid volume excess related to sodium and water retention

DESIRED PATIENT OUTCOME

The patient will maintain adequate fluid balance

Outcome measurement criteria

- ☐ Balanced fluid intake and output
- ☐ Weight within acceptable range
- ☐ Vital signs within normal ranges
- ☐ Absence of oliguria or anuria
- ☐ Absence of peripheral edema
- ☐ Decrease in neck vein distention
- ☐ Return of blood urea nitrogen (BUN) and serum creatinine to baseline levels
- ☐ Serum electrolyte levels within normal ranges

Key interventions

- Measure vital signs at least every 4 hours.
- Assess breath sounds, and check for peripheral edema and jugular vein distention to detect changes in fluid status.
- Monitor 24-hour fluid intake and output. Report significant imbalances to the physician.

- Administer diuretics, as prescribed, and monitor the patient's response.
- Weigh the patient daily.
- Maintain fluid restrictions, as ordered.
- Monitor BUN and serum creatinine and electrolyte levels daily, and report significant changes to the physician. Take special note of serum potassium level, which reveals the patient's response to diuretics.

NURSING DIAGNOSIS

Altered nutrition: less than body requirements related to nausea, vomiting, and dietary restrictions

DESIRED PATIENT OUTCOME

The patient will maintain adequate nutritional intake

Outcome measurement criteria

- ☐ Maintenance of acceptable weight
- ☐ Adequate fluid intake and output
- ☐ Verbalization of relief from nausea and vomiting
- ☐ Serum calcium, lipid, potassium, and protein levels within normal ranges
- ☐ Adherence to dietary restrictions

Key interventions

- Monitor fluid intake and output.
- Weigh the patient daily.
- Observe for nausea and vomiting.
- Administer antiemetic agents, as needed and prescribed, and monitor the patient's response.
- Offer ginger ale and other effervescent soft drinks, as tolerated, within fluid restrictions.

- Provide calories in form of carbohydrates and fats.
- Explain importance of avoiding protein and potassium intake until BUN and serum potassium levels start to fall.
- Perform frequent oral hygiene to eliminate unpleasant tastes.
- Monitor serum calcium, lipid, potassium, and protein levels, and report significant changes to the physician.
- Consult the dietitian for evaluation of complex nutritional problems.

NURSING DIAGNOSIS

High risk for injury related to sensorimotor deficits, seizures, and bleeding secondary to nitrogenous waste retention

DESIRED PATIENT OUTCOME

The patient will remain free from injury during hospitalization

Outcome measurement criteria

☐ Absence of signs and symptoms of injury

☐ Absence of seizures

☐ Absence of evidence of unusual bleeding or bruising

☐ Orientation to person, place, and time

☐ Consistent use of call bell for assistance

Key interventions

- Assess level of consciousness.
- Reorient the patient to surroundings, as needed. Involve the family in reorientation.
- Place clock and calendar within the patient's sight.

- Monitor for seizures. Maintain seizure precautions per hospital protocol.
- Keep bed in low position with side rails up to help prevent injury.
- Check for unusual bruising and bleeding from gums and nose.
- Perform guaiac tests on stools and emesis, and report presence of blood to the physician.
- Administer stool softeners, as needed, to prevent bleeding caused by straining at stool.
- Enforce bed rest during acute phase of illness.
- Assess motor skills, and monitor ambulation as the patient's condition improves.
- Instruct the patient to use soft toothbrush and electric razor to prevent bleeding associated with impaired coagulation.
- Explain how to use call bell to the patient and family, and encourage its consistent use.

NURSING DIAGNOSIS

High risk for infection related to diminished immune response

DESIRED PATIENT OUTCOME

The patient will remain free of infection

Outcome measurement criteria

- ☐ Oral temperature at or below 99.0° F (37.2° C)
- ☐ Vital signs within normal ranges
- ☐ Absence of signs and symptoms of infection
- ☐ White blood cell (WBC) count within normal range
- ☐ Absence of diaphoresis and chills

☐ Demonstration of adequate hygiene practices

Key interventions

- Measure oral temperature every 4 hours.
- Monitor WBC count, and report significant changes to the physician.
- Observe for diaphoresis and chills.
- Maintain strict asepsis during invasive procedures and wound care.
- Assist with coughing, deep breathing, and turning to prevent respiratory tract infections and skin breakdown.
- Administer antipruritic agents, as prescribed, to minimize itching.
- Assess skin daily for scratches.
- Provide meticulous skin care, including daily baths with moisturizing soap to combat dry skin.
- Teach the patient and family proper handwashing technique.
- Advise the patient to avoid exposure to people with infections.

NURSING DIAGNOSIS

Knowledge deficit regarding follow-up care necessary to prevent disease recurrences

DESIRED PATIENT OUTCOME

The patient will express an understanding of necessary follow-up care

Outcome measurement criteria

☐ Identification of causes of acute renal failure

☐ Verbalization of fluid and dietary restrictions

☐ Demonstration of correct technique for measuring pulse rate, blood pressure, and fluid intake and output

☐ Verbalization of prescribed medication regimen

☐ Verbalization of understanding of dialysis, if applicable

Key interventions

- Explain causes of acute renal failure.
- Discuss usual changes in renal function after acute episodes.
- Explain fluid and dietary restrictions.
- Teach the patient how to measure heart rate, blood pressure, and fluid intake and output.
- Discuss signs and symptoms of infection and recurrence of acute renal failure. Instruct the patient to report these to the physician immediately.
- Review names, purposes, dosages, and common adverse effects of prescribed medications.
- Describe dialysis procedure, if applicable.
- Emphasize need to control hypertension and avoid nephrotoxic drugs.
- Advise the patient to follow discharge instructions scrupulously.

Chronic renal failure

Slow, irreversible impairment of renal function caused by such conditions as hypertensive or diabetic nephropathy, glomerulonephritis, and polycystic kidney disease.

NURSING DIAGNOSIS

Altered renal tissue perfusion related to irreversible kidney damage

DESIRED PATIENT OUTCOME

The patient will exhibit improved renal tissue perfusion

Outcome measurement criteria

- ☐ Blood pressure below 160/100 mm Hg
- ☐ Adequate urine output
- ☐ Decrease in edema
- ☐ Balanced fluid intake and output
- ☐ Maintenance of acceptable weight
- ☐ Absence of mental status changes
- ☐ Blood urea nitrogen (BUN) and serum creatinine and electrolyte levels within expected ranges
- ☐ Arterial blood gas (ABG) values within expected ranges
- ☐ Hemoglobin and hematocrit values within normal ranges
- ☐ Electrocardiogram (ECG) within normal limits
- ☐ Respiratory rate and depth within normal ranges

Key interventions

- Assess mental status every 8 hours.

- Check for edema, crackles, and neck vein distention to help evaluate fluid status.
- Weigh the patient daily.
- Monitor hemoglobin and hematocrit values.
- Monitor fluid intake and output. Evaluate fluid balance every 24 hours, and report significant imbalances to the physician.
- Review ABG values, and assess for changes in respiratory rate and depth, which may indicate acidosis.
- Monitor sitting and standing blood pressure every 4 hours to detect hypotension.
- Monitor BUN and serum creatinine, potassium, and sodium levels to help assess renal function.
- Monitor ECG for arrhythmias associated with serum potassium imbalance.
- Administer medications, as prescribed, and monitor the patient's response. Be aware that impaired kidney function may necessitate adjustment of drug dosages and administration schedules.
- Offer restricted fluid intake over entire 24-hour period to prevent nocturnal dehydration.

NURSING DIAGNOSIS

High risk for impaired skin integrity related to dry, itchy skin secondary to uremia

DESIRED PATIENT OUTCOME

The patient's skin will remain intact

Outcome measurement criteria

☐ Absence of skin breakdown, excoriation, and scratches

☐ Absence of itching

☐ Adequate skin lubrication

☐ Absence of signs of skin infection

☐ Decrease in edema

Key interventions

- Assess skin for excessive dryness, excoriation, and signs of infection. Check skin folds and edematous areas closely.
- Administer antipruritic medications, as prescribed, and document the patient's response.
- Observe for discomfort and itching.
- Reposition the patient every 2 hours to prevent pressure-related skin breakdown.
- Keep the patient's skin clean and dry, and moisturize it with lotion and oil. Add vinegar to bath water to ease itching.
- Maintain room at comfortable temperature to prevent heat-related discomfort.
- Trim the patient's fingernails to prevent scratches.

NURSING DIAGNOSIS

Altered nutrition: less than body requirements related to nausea, vomiting, and anorexia

DESIRED PATIENT OUTCOME

The patient will maintain adequate nutritional intake

Outcome measurement criteria

☐ Adequate fluid intake and output

☐ Maintenance of acceptable weight

☐ Verbalization of relief from nausea and vomiting

- ☐ Serum calcium, lipid, potassium, and protein levels within normal ranges
- ☐ Positive nitrogen balance
- ☐ Adherence to dietary restrictions

Key interventions

- Monitor fluid intake and output.
- Weigh the patient daily.
- Observe for nausea and vomiting.
- Monitor serum calcium, lipid, potassium, and protein levels, and report significant changes to the physician.
- Administer antiemetic medications, as needed and prescribed, and document the patient's response.
- Provide preferred foods, attractively presented, to enhance appetite. Make sure calories come from carbohydrates and fats, not proteins.
- Offer ginger ale and other effervescent soft drinks, as tolerated, within fluid restrictions.
- Explain importance of avoiding protein and potassium intake until serum potassium and BUN levels start to fall.
- Perform frequent oral hygiene. Offer sugarless gum or hard candy to eliminate unpleasant tastes.
- Consult the dietitian for evaluation of complex nutritional problems.

NURSING DIAGNOSIS

High risk for altered thought processes related to uremia

DESIRED PATIENT OUTCOME

The patient will maintain orientation to person, place, and time

Outcome measurement criteria

- ☐ Orientation to person, place, and time
- ☐ Absence of behavioral and personality changes
- ☐ Absence of seizures
- ☐ Absence of signs and symptoms of injury

Key interventions

- Assess neurologic status, including level of consciousness.
- Monitor for behavioral and personality changes.
- Reorient the patient to surroundings frequently. Involve the family in reorientation.
- Place clock and calendar within the patient's sight.
- Keep bed in low position with side rails up to help prevent injury.
- Place call bell within the patient's reach.
- Observe for seizures, and implement seizure precautions, as needed.
- Discuss the patient's sleep and rest patterns, which may be altered by uremia.
- Maintain calm, rational approach. Give the patient ample time to respond to questions because uremia may affect short-term memory.

NURSING DIAGNOSIS

Powerlessness related to effects of chronic illness on lifestyle

DESIRED PATIENT OUTCOME

The patient will express a sense of regained control over health situation

Outcome measurement criteria

☐ Verbalization of concerns and fears about health status

☐ Participation in care and treatment decisions

☐ Participation in self-care activities, as tolerated

☐ Verbalization of feelings of having regained control over health situation

☐ Verbalization of acceptance of required lifestyle changes

☐ Use of effective strategies to reduce anxiety and manage chronic illness

Key interventions

- Encourage the patient to express feelings.
- Allow time to discuss the patient's concerns and fears.
- Maintain nonjudgmental approach, and avoid responding defensively. Accept that feelings of powerlessness are normal in patients with chronic illness.
- Offer reassurance when feelings of powerlessness arise.
- Encourage the patient to perform self-care activities, as tolerated.
- Allow the patient to participate in care and treatment decisions.
- Urge the family to support the patient without being controlling.
- Make sure the patient's spiritual needs are being met. Contact the hospital chaplain or clergyperson of choice, if appropriate.
- Refer the patient and family to other services, as appropriate, to help resolve problems.

NURSING DIAGNOSIS

High risk for ineffective management of therapeutic regimen related to complex nature of disease

DESIRED PATIENT OUTCOME

The patient will develop a plan for integrating the therapeutic regimen into daily life

Outcome measurement criteria

- ☐ Identification of causes of chronic renal failure
- ☐ Adherence to fluid and dietary restrictions
- ☐ Adherence to prescribed medication regimen
- ☐ Verbalization of understanding of dialysis, if applicable
- ☐ Demonstration of correct techniques for measuring pulse rate, blood pressure, and fluid intake and output

Key interventions

- Describe nature and stages of chronic renal failure.
- Discuss fluid and dietary restrictions.
- Explain how fluid and dietary restrictions affect blood chemistry results.
- Teach correct techniques for measuring pulse rate, blood pressure, and fluid intake and output.
- Explain reasons for changes in skin color and texture. Encourage good hygiene to minimize itching.
- Advise the patient to rest between activities to minimize fatigue.
- Instruct the patient to avoid exposure to people with infections.
- Instruct the patient to report vital sign changes, extreme fatigue, decreased urine output, and signs and symptoms of urinary tract infection to the physician.
- Review names, purposes, dosages, and common adverse effects of prescribed medications.
- Explain dialysis procedure, if applicable.
- Stress the need to follow discharge instructions.

Hemodialysis

Procedure in which wastes or impurities are removed from the patient's blood through semipermeable membrane for diffusion and ultrafiltration and then returned to the circulation; used to treat various renal and toxic conditions.

NURSING DIAGNOSIS

High risk for fluid volume deficit related to fluid removal during dialysis and possible blood loss from access device

DESIRED PATIENT OUTCOME

The patient will maintain adequate fluid balance

Outcome measurement criteria

☐ Balanced fluid intake and output

☐ Blood pressure within normal range

☐ Stable heart and respiratory rates

☐ Absence of tachycardia, dizziness, restlessness, nausea, and vomiting

☐ Clotting time within normal range

☐ Acceptable weight loss without hypotension

☐ Absence of blood loss from access device

Key interventions

- Assess vital signs before and during dialysis to establish baseline measurements and help detect changes in fluid status.
- Weigh the patient before and after dialysis, and document results.

- Contact the physician to clarify withholding of drugs that may contribute to hypovolemia, such as analgesics, hypnotic agents, tranquilizers, and nitroglycerin. Unless the patient has severe hypertension, withhold rapid-acting antihypertensive drugs on morning of dialysis, as ordered.
- Observe for signs and symptoms of hypovolemia, such as dizziness, restlessness, anxiety, nausea, vomiting, and postural hypotension.
- Evaluate clotting time to monitor effectiveness of anticoagulant therapy.
- Assess patency of fistula or graft used for dialysis by palpating or auscultating for bruit. Check patency of external shunt by observing for continuous blood flow through shunt.
- Apply pressure dressing to fistula site, and monitor frequently for bleeding or oozing.
- Observe closely for signs and symptoms of bleeding in response to anticoagulants.
- Avoid I.M. injections and venipuncture during and shortly after dialysis.

NURSING DIAGNOSIS

High risk for infection related to invasive nature of hemodialysis

DESIRED PATIENT OUTCOME

The patient will remain free of infection

Outcome measurement criteria

☐ Oral temperature at or below 99.0° F (37.2° C)

☐ White blood cell (WBC) count within normal range

☐ Vital signs within normal ranges

- ☐ Absence of diaphoresis and chills
- ☐ Absence of warmth, redness, tenderness, and swelling at graft, shunt, or fistula site

Key interventions

- Measure oral temperature and other vital signs at least every 4 hours.
- Observe for diaphoresis and chills.
- Monitor WBC count, and report increases to the physician. Be aware that even slight elevations in temperature and WBC count may reflect significant infection.
- Use sterile technique when inserting and removing access needle.
- Check graft, shunt, or fistula site for signs and symptoms of infection, including redness, warmth, tenderness, and swelling.
- Maintain universal precautions at all times to protect the patient and nurse from spread of infection.

NURSING DIAGNOSIS

Altered thought processes related to disequilibrium syndrome secondary to hemodialysis

DESIRED PATIENT OUTCOME

The patient will remain free of signs and symptoms of disequilibrium syndrome

Outcome measurement criteria

- ☐ Vital signs within normal ranges
- ☐ Orientation to person, place, and time
- ☐ Absence of headache, restlessness, nausea, and vomiting
- ☐ Absence of seizures

☐ Absence of signs and symptoms of injury

Key interventions

- Measure vital signs frequently to detect changes.
- Monitor for confusion, headache, nausea, vomiting, and restlessness.
- Observe the patient closely toward end of dialysis session and afterward, when disequilibrium syndrome is most likely to occur.
- Implement seizure precautions, if necessary. Report seizures or unusual behavior to the physician immediately.
- Keep bed in low position with side rails up to prevent injury. Keep call bell within the patient's reach at all times.
- Administer mild analgesic, as prescribed, if the patient complains of headache.
- Provide quiet, restful environment. Keep lights dim, and maintain comfortable ambient temperature.
- Collaborate with the physician to keep initial hemodialysis sessions short and at frequent intervals to avoid drastic blood chemistry changes, which may lead to disequilibrium syndrome.

NURSING DIAGNOSIS

Altered family processes related to the patient's dependence on hemodialysis

DESIRED PATIENT OUTCOME

The patient and family members will exhibit adaptive coping mechanisms

Outcome measurement criteria

- ☐ Verbalization by each family member of changing roles within family
- ☐ Verbalization of acceptance of feelings regarding changing roles
- ☐ Identification of family member who will act as head of household, if appropriate
- ☐ Assumption by other family members of duties normally carried out by the patient
- ☐ Identification of support systems and community resources

Key interventions

- Observe interactions among family members.
- Discuss implications of dialysis with the patient and family. Encourage them to discuss concerns and feelings.
- Encourage the family to appoint one member to act as head of household, if appropriate.
- Offer emotional support to the patient and family regarding changing roles and expectations.
- Provide the patient and family with accurate information needed to make decisions about care, treatment, and patient's dependence on dialysis.
- Arrange for and participate in family conferences, if appropriate.
- Help the family identify support systems and determine which ones to use.
- Provide the family with list of community resources.
- Contact the social services department for additional counseling and referral, as needed.

NURSING DIAGNOSIS

Knowledge deficit regarding dialysis and follow-up care

DESIRED PATIENT OUTCOME

The patient will express an understanding of dialysis and follow-up care

Outcome measurement criteria

- ☐ Verbalization of understanding of dialysis
- ☐ Adherence to dietary restrictions
- ☐ Adherence to prescribed medication regimen
- ☐ Demonstration of correct technique for shunt, fistula, or graft care
- ☐ Identification of conditions to report to the physician
- ☐ Verbalization of importance of follow-up care

Key interventions

- Explain need for dialysis and its effects on kidney function, blood chemistry results, and dietary restrictions.
- Describe sequence of activities that occur during dialysis.
- Discuss common complications of hemodialysis, such as hypotension, cramps, nausea, and vomiting. Explain how these problems are treated.
- Review prescribed diet, including restricted intake of protein, potassium, sodium, and fluids. Ask the dietitian for help, if necessary.
- Discuss names, purposes, dosages, and common adverse effects of prescribed medications. If ordered, instruct the patient to withhold certain drugs before dialysis sessions.
- Demonstrate how to care for vascular access device.

Observe return demonstration.

- Teach the patient how to palpate and auscultate for bruits in shunt or fistula.
- Instruct the patient to report signs and symptoms of infection immediately.
- Teach the patient and family how to control hemorrhage.
- Caution the patient to avoid injections, venipunctures, and blood pressure measurements in arm with vascular access device.
- Advise the patient to avoid practices that would constrict shunt or fistula, such as sleeping on affected arm and wearing tight clothing.

Nephrectomy

Surgical removal of kidney performed to remove a tumor or to treat other diseases or injury.

NURSING DIAGNOSIS

High risk for fluid volume deficit related to surgery

DESIRED PATIENT OUTCOME

The patient will maintain adequate fluid balance

Outcome measurement criteria

- ☐ Urine output of at least 30 ml/hour
- ☐ Adequate I.V. or oral fluid intake
- ☐ Vital signs within normal ranges
- ☐ Absence of excessive bleeding from incision
- ☐ Maintenance of hemodynamic stability
- ☐ Hemoglobin and hematocrit values within normal ranges
- ☐ Urine specific gravity within normal range
- ☐ Serum electrolyte levels within normal ranges

Key interventions

- Measure vital signs every 4 hours. Stay alert for evidence of fluid volume depletion, such as decreasing blood pressure and weak, thready pulse.
- Provide adequate hydration through I.V. and oral routes, as ordered.
- Monitor and document fluid intake and output.

- Observe for signs and symptoms of shock, including pallor and cool, clammy skin.
- Assess surgical dressing frequently for excessive drainage and bleeding. Reinforce dressing, as needed, and notify the physician of excessive drainage or bleeding.
- Monitor for changes in level of consciousness.
- Measure urine specific gravity at least every 8 hours. Report significant changes to the physician.
- Monitor hemoglobin, hematocrit, and serum electrolyte values daily, and report significant changes to the physician.

NURSING DIAGNOSIS

Pain related to location of incision

DESIRED PATIENT OUTCOME

The patient will experience relief from pain

Outcome measurement criteria

- ☐ Verbalization of adequate pain relief
- ☐ Vital signs within normal ranges
- ☐ Participation in self-care activities, as tolerated
- ☐ Relaxed facial expression and muscle tone

Key interventions

- Ask the patient to describe nature, location, and severity of pain.
- Determine how pain affects the patient's mental state, appetite, and activity level.
- Explain concept of postoperative pain management, including meaning of *p.r.n.*

- Administer pain medication, as prescribed, before activities. Evaluate effectiveness of medication.
- Encourage the patient to request pain medication before pain becomes severe.
- Monitor for respiratory depression and other adverse effects of narcotics, if prescribed.
- Discuss use of patient-controlled analgesia (PCA). Teach the patient how to use PCA pump, if applicable, and observe return demonstration.
- Reassure the patient and family that postoperative narcotic addiction is rare.
- Switch to oral analgesics, as ordered, once pain subsides and the patient can tolerate oral intake.
- Consult the physician and clinical pharmacist if pain management is ineffective.

NURSING DIAGNOSIS

Ineffective breathing pattern related to location of incision and narcotic analgesics

DESIRED PATIENT OUTCOME

The patient will maintain an effective breathing pattern

Outcome measurement criteria

- ☐ Respiratory rate of 12 to 20 breaths/minute
- ☐ Absence of adventitious lung sounds
- ☐ Arterial blood gas (ABG) or pulse oximetry values within normal ranges
- ☐ Normal skin color
- ☐ Absence of pneumonia and atelectasis
- ☐ Verbalization of increasing breathing comfort

- ☐ Demonstration of correct techniques for coughing, deep breathing, splinting, and using incentive spirometer
- ☐ Demonstration of ability to expectorate pulmonary secretions

Key interventions

- Assess respiratory status every 4 hours, noting adventitious lung sounds.
- Observe for splinting, shallow breathing, and dyspnea.
- Measure vital signs frequently.
- Encourage the patient to turn, cough, and deep-breathe every 2 hours.
- Teach the patient how to splint incision, and observe return demonstration.
- Assist the patient with activities of daily living and ambulation during immediate postoperative period.
- Monitor ABG or pulse oximetry values. Report significant changes to the physician.

NURSING DIAGNOSIS

High risk for infection related to disruption in tissue integrity

DESIRED PATIENT OUTCOME

The patient will remain free of infection

Outcome measurement criteria

- ☐ Oral temperature at or below 99.0° F (37.2° C)
- ☐ White blood cell (WBC) count within normal range
- ☐ Absence of erythema, purulent drainage, and tenderness at incision site

- ☐ Approximation of wound edges
- ☐ Negative blood and wound cultures

Key interventions

- Measure oral temperature at least every 4 hours.
- Observe for chills, fever, diaphoresis, and changes in vital signs.
- Assess wound at each shift for signs and symptoms of infection, such as warmth, redness, drainage, tenderness, and odor.
- Monitor WBC count, and report significant increases to the physician.
- Obtain blood and wound cultures, as needed, and monitor results.
- Consult the infection control practitioner, as needed.

NURSING DIAGNOSIS

Impaired health maintenance management related to lack of information about follow-up care

DESIRED PATIENT OUTCOME

The patient will express an understanding of follow-up care

Outcome measurement criteria

- ☐ Demonstration of correct wound care technique
- ☐ Verbalization of activity limitations
- ☐ Verbalization of signs and symptoms of infection
- ☐ Identification of conditions to report to the primary health care practitioner
- ☐ Verbalization of prescribed medication regimen
- ☐ Identification of available community resources

Key interventions

- Teach the patient and family how to perform wound care. Observe several return demonstrations to verify mastery.
- Discuss activity restrictions, such as refraining from heavy lifting for 8 weeks.
- Emphasize need to avoid vigorous exercise and contact sports.
- Instruct the patient to report redness, warmth, pain, swelling, or drainage at incision site.
- Advise the patient to report signs and symptoms of urinary tract infection to the primary health care practitioner immediately.
- Review names, purposes, dosages, and common adverse effects of prescribed drugs.
- Teach the patient to wear seat belt when traveling to prevent injury to remaining kidney.
- Provide information about available community resources.
- Consult the social services department for home care assistance if the patient cannot perform self-care activities.

Urinary diversion

Alternative route to establish unimpeded urine flow via stoma, created surgically using segment of small intestine; permanent urinary diversions include ureterostomy, ileal conduit, and continent urinary diversion.

NURSING DIAGNOSIS

Fear related to lack of information about surgery and presence of urinary diversion

DESIRED PATIENT OUTCOME

The patient will exhibit decreased fear

Outcome measurement criteria

- ☐ Relaxed facial expression and muscle tone
- ☐ Verbalization of concerns and fears about surgery
- ☐ Verbalization of understanding of purpose of surgery
- ☐ Discussion of expected surgical outcome
- ☐ Verbalization of decreased fear within 1 week after surgery
- ☐ Demonstration of proper handling of urostomy appliance, if applicable

Key interventions

- Encourage the patient to discuss concerns and fears about surgery and urinary diversion.
- Assess the patient's willingness to learn about surgery and urinary diversion.
- Explain that the patient will undergo bowel preparation before surgery.

- Advise the patient to consume low-residue diet 2 days before surgery, followed by clear liquids on day before surgery.
- Show the patient and family where urostomy will be located, using diagrams and models.
- Describe expected appearance of stoma.
- Show urine-collection appliance to the patient, if applicable.
- Emphasize that surgery will not necessitate significant changes in work routine, activity level, diet, clothing, or hobbies.
- Provide reassurance that the staff will help the patient master stoma care before discharge.
- Ask if the patient would like to talk to someone who has undergone same procedure.
- Consult the enterostomal therapist for additional instructions.

NURSING DIAGNOSIS

Altered urinary elimination related to urinary diversion

DESIRED PATIENT OUTCOME

The patient will maintain adequate urine output

Outcome measurement criteria

- ☐ Adequate urine output
- ☐ Normal stoma color
- ☐ Absence of edema around stoma
- ☐ Absence of blood in urine by 3rd day after surgery

Key interventions

- Monitor amount and color of urine. Expect blood in

urine for first 2 days after surgery.

- Evaluate stoma and suture line for edema, necrosis, and signs of infection. Report significant findings to the physician.
- Connect stoma pouch to bedside drainage collection device during immediate postoperative period.
- Keep drainage tubes free of kinks to ensure patency.
- Check drainage sites for urinary drainage if stoma output diminishes. Be aware that diminished stoma output indicates ileal-ureteral leakage or decreased renal function.
- Consult the enterostomal therapist to ensure adequacy of pouching system.

NURSING DIAGNOSIS

High risk for impaired skin integrity related to urine leakage around stoma

DESIRED PATIENT OUTCOME

The patient will maintain skin integrity around stoma

Outcome measurement criteria

- ☐ Absence of tenderness, irritation, and redness around stoma
- ☐ Properly fitting stoma pouch
- ☐ Absence of signs of tape rash
- ☐ Urine pH of 6.0 or lower
- ☐ Demonstration of correct skin care technique

Key interventions

- Assess skin around stoma frequently for irritation, redness, ulceration, and rash.

- Monitor urine pH during each shift.
- Clean skin around stoma with mild soap and water to remove urine and mucus secretions. Allow skin to dry thoroughly.
- Apply skin barrier to irritated skin.
- Center pouch over stoma, and then press pouch into place and hold for 30 seconds to bond adhesive. Eliminate wrinkles or creases, which may cause leaks.
- Explain all procedures to the patient and family.
- Provide step-by-step instructions on how to change stoma pouch and care for surrounding skin. Observe return demonstrations.
- Consult the enterostomal therapist for additional instructions and follow-up care.

NURSING DIAGNOSIS

Body image disturbance related to presence of stoma and external pouch

DESIRED PATIENT OUTCOME

The patient will adapt to presence of stoma and external pouch

Outcome measurement criteria

- ☐ Verbalization of feelings about stoma and pouch
- ☐ Direct observation of stoma site
- ☐ Participation in self-care activities
- ☐ Verbalization of positive feelings about self
- ☐ Use of appropriate strategies to cope with altered body image

Key interventions

- Assess the patient's attitude toward stoma and pouch. Note denial, anger, or embarrassment.
- Encourage the patient to discuss feelings.
- Stress that pouch cannot be detected under most clothing.
- Teach the patient how to manage leaks and odor problems.
- Encourage the patient and family to ask questions.
- Explain all procedures associated with stoma and pouch.
- Ask if the patient would like to talk to someone else who has stoma and external pouch.
- Refer the patient and family to appropriate community resources and counseling services, as needed.

NURSING DIAGNOSIS

Altered health maintenance related to lack of information about urostomy

DESIRED PATIENT OUTCOME

The patient will express adequate understanding of urostomy care and follow-up care

Outcome measurement criteria

- ☐ Discussion of urostomy care
- ☐ Demonstration of correct pouch-changing technique
- ☐ Demonstration of correct skin care technique
- ☐ Identification of foods that cause urine odor
- ☐ Verbalization of fluid intake guidelines
- ☐ Demonstration of correct urine pH monitoring technique

- ☐ Identification of local urostomy supplier
- ☐ Identification of community resources

Key interventions

- Offer verbal and written information about urostomy.
- Teach the patient to empty urostomy bag (pouch) when it is half full.
- Reinforce correct technique for changing pouch and caring for surrounding skin. Observe return demonstrations.
- Teach the patient to measure urine pH on first few drops of urine in fresh pouch.
- Mention that pouch usually can stay in place for 3 to 5 days if it is applied properly.
- Instruct the patient to use drainage bag overnight.
- Teach the patient to use skin barrier to treat minor skin irritation.
- Advise the patient to swab vinegar on stoma if urinary crystals (caused by alkaline urine) begin to form.
- Inform the patient that asparagus, eggs, fish, onions, and spicy foods cause strong urine odor.
- Emphasize importance of drinking 10 to 12 glasses of fluid daily to maintain urine acidity. Advise the patient to limit milk consumption to four glasses daily to avoid raising urine pH.
- Instruct the patient to report markedly decreased urine output, skin ulceration, and signs of localized or systemic infection to the primary health care practitioner.
- Supply names of local suppliers of urostomy products.
- Provide list of community resources, including local chapter of ostomy association.
- Explain importance of seeing the urologist every 6 to 12 months for follow-up care.

Urinary tract infection

Bacterial invasion of one or more structures of urinary tract [UTI], usually by organisms normally found in intestinal tract.

NURSING DIAGNOSIS

Pain related to inflammation of urethra, bladder, or kidneys

DESIRED PATIENT OUTCOME

The patient will experience relief from pain

Outcome measurement criteria

- ☐ Verbalization of adequate pain relief
- ☐ Vital signs within normal ranges
- ☐ Absence of bladder spasms
- ☐ Absence of nausea and vomiting
- ☐ Relaxed facial expression and muscle tone

Key interventions

- Ask the patient to describe pain, including location, duration, and severity, as well as associated symptoms.
- Measure vital signs every 4 hours.
- Administer pain medication, as prescribed, and document the patient's response.
- Administer antispasmodic medication, as prescribed. Advise the patient that this medication may discolor urine.
- Provide sitz baths to decrease pain from urethritis.
- Offer back rubs for short-term pain relief.

- Encourage increased fluid intake to relieve burning sensation associated with lower urinary tract infection (UTI).

NURSING DIAGNOSIS

Ineffective management of therapeutic regimen related to lack of information regarding prevention of recurrent UTIs and need for follow-up care

DESIRED PATIENT OUTCOME

The patient will integrate a program for preventing UTIs into daily living

Outcome measurement criteria

- ☐ Identification of possible causes of UTI
- ☐ Verbalization of signs and symptoms to report
- ☐ Oral temperature at or below 99.0° F (37.2° C)
- ☐ Absence of chills and diaphoresis
- ☐ Clear, nonodorous urine
- ☐ Negative urine cultures
- ☐ Demonstration of adequate fluid intake
- ☐ Identification of measures that help prevent UTI recurrence
- ☐ Use of appropriate hygiene practices
- ☐ Verbalization of prescribed medication regimen

Key interventions

- Determine if the patient experiences recurrent UTIs.
- Help the patient identify common causes of UTI, such as inadequate emptying or overdistention of bladder, poor hygiene, and history of renal calculi.

- Teach the patient to measure temperature. Instruct the patient to stay alert for and report chills, diaphoresis, restlessness, and general discomfort.
- Encourage the patient to drink at least 2,000 ml of fluid daily. Explain that cranberry, plum, and prune juices help prevent UTIs by maintaining urine acidity.
- Teach correct technique for obtaining clean-catch, midstream urine specimen.
- Instruct the patient to check urine for cloudiness, blood, sediment, and strong odor.
- Teach a female patient to wipe from urethral meatus to anal area after voiding to help prevent infection. Instruct her to wear underwear and swimsuits with cotton crotches because synthetic materials trap moisture against perineum, promoting bacterial growth and infection.
- Instruct a female patient to empty her bladder and drink fluids after sexual intercourse to flush out ascending organisms.
- Review names, purposes, dosages, and common adverse effects of prescribed drugs.
- Advise the patient to complete full course of prescribed antibiotic therapy, even if symptoms improve.
- Instruct the patient to follow administration instructions on antibiotic prescription bottle. Encourage yogurt consumption to replace normal intestinal flora lost during antibiotic therapy.
- Advise the patient to report fever, chills, flank pain, or urinary frequency, burning, or pain to the primary health care practitioner immediately.

Urolithiasis

Formation of mineral crystals (commonly called kidney stones or urinary calculi) in urinary tract.

NURSING DIAGNOSIS

Pain related to spasms and anoxia of ureter wall secondary to renal calculi

DESIRED PATIENT OUTCOME

The patient will experience relief from pain

Outcome measurement criteria

- ☐ Verbalization of adequate pain relief
- ☐ Vital signs within normal ranges
- ☐ Absence of nausea and vomiting
- ☐ Relaxed facial expression and muscle tone

Key interventions

- Ask the patient to describe pain, including its location, duration, and severity.
- Measure vital signs every 4 hours.
- Administer analgesics and antiemetics, as prescribed, and monitor the patient's response.
- Apply heat to painful areas for 15 to 20 minutes every 2 hours.
- Observe for nausea, vomiting, and associated signs and symptoms.

NURSING DIAGNOSIS

Altered urinary elimination related to pain and possible urinary tract obstruction secondary to renal calculi

DESIRED PATIENT OUTCOME

The patient will regain normal urinary elimination

Outcome measurement criteria

- ☐ Adequate urine output
- ☐ Fluid intake of 2,000 to 3,000 ml daily
- ☐ Absence of dysuria and hematuria
- ☐ Blood urea nitrogen (BUN) and serum creatinine levels within normal ranges
- ☐ Urine pH of 6.0 or lower

Key interventions

- Measure and strain urine at each voiding, and observe urine for color, sediment, blood, and calculi. Report significant findings or urine output less than 30 ml/hour to the physician.
- Encourage the patient to drink 2,000 to 3,000 ml of fluid daily, unless contraindicated.
- Monitor and document fluid intake and output.
- Test urine pH each shift.
- Administer antibiotics, as prescribed, to maintain therapeutic blood levels.
- Monitor BUN and serum creatinine and electrolyte levels to ensure early detection of renal dysfunction.
- Observe for signs and symptoms of urinary tract infection, including flank pain, bladder spasms, fever, chills, urinary frequency, and dysuria.

NURSING DIAGNOSIS

Altered health maintenance related to lack of knowledge about preventing renal calculi recurrence

DESIRED PATIENT OUTCOME

The patient will verbalize an understanding of ways to prevent renal calculi recurrence

Outcome measurement criteria

- ☐ Verbalization of dietary restrictions
- ☐ Verbalization of need for increased fluid intake
- ☐ Discussion of importance of physical activity
- ☐ Demonstration of correct technique for measuring and interpreting urine pH
- ☐ Identification of signs and symptoms of renal calculi recurrence

Key interventions

- Instruct the patient to limit intake of foods high in calculus-forming substances, such as dairy products; green, leafy vegetables; meat; whole grains; chocolate; and caffeine.
- Advise the patient to drink 2,000 to 3,000 ml of fluid daily.
- Encourage regular activity to decrease urinary stasis.
- Teach correct technique for measuring and interpreting urine pH.
- Instruct the patient to report pain, hematuria, and oliguria to the primary health care practitioner immediately.

Breast cancer and mastectomy

Breast cancer is the uncontrolled growth of neoplastic cells in breast; may be classified as adenocarcinoma, intraductal, infiltrating, lobular carcinoma in situ, inflammatory, or circumscribed. Treatment may involve mastectomy—surgical removal of all or part of affected breast, possibly with removal of chest muscles and axillary lymph nodes.

NURSING DIAGNOSIS

Decisional conflict (treatment options) related to lack of information

DESIRED PATIENT OUTCOME

The patient will make an informed decision about treatment options

Outcome measurement criteria

- ☐ Verbalization of feelings about current health situation
- ☐ Identification of personal strengths
- ☐ Discussion of conflicts related to treatment options
- ☐ Discussion of consequences of various treatment options
- ☐ Participation in minor decisions about daily care
- ☐ Verbalization of increased comfort in making treatment decisions
- ☐ Acceptance of help from family, friends, and clergy

Key interventions

- Encourage the patient to discuss concerns and feelings. Provide uninterrupted time to listen.
- Acknowledge the patient's values and beliefs as well as present decisional conflict.
- Assist the patient with identifying physical, psychological, intellectual, and spiritual strengths.
- Provide accurate information about breast cancer.
- Help the patient identify available treatment options. Discuss possible consequences of each option. Encourage her to ask questions, and clarify any misconceptions.
- Encourage and assist the patient in making minor decisions about daily care, to promote autonomy and confidence in decision making.
- Support use of religious practices and rituals during hospitalization, if patient uses these. Contact the chaplain or the patient's clergy, as requested.
- Encourage the patient to accept emotional support from family, friends, and clergy to gain comfort and strength.
- Demonstrate acceptance and support of the patient's decision about treatment options.

NURSING DIAGNOSIS

Fear related to uncertain course of disease and treatment

DESIRED PATIENT OUTCOME

The patient will exhibit decreased fear

Outcome measurement criteria

- ☐ Verbalization of decreased fear
- ☐ Vital signs within normal ranges
- ☐ Relaxed facial expression and muscle tone

☐ Use of relaxation techniques to help control fear

Key interventions

- Assess for signs and symptoms of anxiety and fear.
- Determine source of the patient's fear by listening to concerns. Clarify any misconceptions and answer questions honestly.
- Listen for verbal cues indicating an increase or decrease in fear.
- Explain all preoperative and postoperative care.
- Teach relaxation techniques, such as deep breathing, music therapy, and guided imagery.
- Maintain environment conducive to relaxation.

NURSING DIAGNOSIS

Fluid volume excess related to impaired lymphatic drainage and surgery

DESIRED PATIENT OUTCOME

The patient will experience minimal lymphedema

Outcome measurement criteria

☐ Little or no increase in circumference of affected arm

☐ Absence of neurovascular changes in affected arm

☐ Serum albumin and sodium values within normal ranges

☐ Little or no evidence of edema

☐ Absence of skin breakdown

☐ Performance of required exercises

Key interventions

- Before surgery, measure circumference of each arm 2½"

above and below elbow, to establish baseline.

- After surgery, measure circumference of each arm daily. Report increase in circumference of affected arm to the physician.
- Monitor serum albumin and sodium levels, and report significant changes to the physician.
- Apply antiembolism sleeve to affected arm, as ordered.
- Use mechanical pressure pump, as ordered, if lymphedema is severe.
- Elevate affected arm on pillow, with elbow above shoulder and wrist above elbow.
- Monitor neurovascular status of affected arm each shift. Report pulse deficit.
- Assess arm for edema by pressing thumb into skin for 5 to 10 seconds. Remove thumb, then observe for depression.
- Observe skin for color, temperature, and degree of translucency.
- Place the patient on air mattress, and pad side rails to protect arm from trauma.
- Instruct the patient not to wear identification band, watch, or other jewelry on affected arm.
- Place sign over the patient's bed to alert health care providers not to draw blood, give injections, or take blood pressure measurements in the affected arm.
- Massage affected arm with lotion, starting at wrist and moving toward shoulder, to increase lymph flow.
- Instruct the patient to perform exercises, as ordered, to prevent muscle deformity, contractures, stiffness, and frozen shoulder.

NURSING DIAGNOSIS

Pain related to surgery

DESIRED PATIENT OUTCOME

The patient will experience relief from pain

Outcome measurement criteria

- ☐ Verbalization of relief from pain
- ☐ Vital signs within normal ranges
- ☐ Relaxed facial expression and muscle tone
- ☐ Participation in self-care activities
- ☐ Demonstration of correct technique for operating patient-controlled analgesia (PCA) pump, if applicable

Key interventions

- Ask the patient to describe nature, location, and severity of pain.
- Explain principles of postoperative pain management, including meaning of *p.r.n.*
- Reassure the patient and family that postoperative narcotic addiction is rare.
- Encourage the patient to request medication before pain becomes severe.
- Administer pain medication, as prescribed, before activities.
- Discuss use of PCA. As appropriate, teach the patient how to use PCA pump, and observe return demonstration.
- Switch to oral analgesics once pain diminishes and the patient can tolerate oral feedings.
- Evaluate effectiveness of pain medication.
- Consult the physician or clinical pharmacist if pain management is ineffective.

NURSING DIAGNOSIS

High risk for infection related to disruption in skin integrity and impaired lymphatic function

DESIRED PATIENT OUTCOME

The patient will remain free of infection during hospitalization

Outcome measurement criteria

- ☐ Oral temperature at or below 99.0° F (37.2° C)
- ☐ White blood cell (WBC) count within normal range
- ☐ Absence of erythema, purulent drainage, and tenderness at incision site

Key interventions

- Measure oral temperature at least every 4 hours.
- Observe for chills, fever, diaphoresis, and changes in vital signs.
- Monitor WBC count for increases indicating infection. Report significant findings to the physician.
- Assess wound each shift for redness, warmth, drainage, tenderness, and odor.
- Monitor all drains for evidence of infection.
- Obtain blood and wound cultures as needed, and monitor results.
- Consult the infection control practitioner, as needed.

NURSING DIAGNOSIS

Body image disturbance related to loss of breast and adverse effects of chemotherapy or radiation therapy

DESIRED PATIENT OUTCOME

The patient will begin to adapt to body image changes during hospitalization

Outcome measurement criteria

- ☐ Identification of body image changes
- ☐ Verbalization of feelings about body image changes
- ☐ Verbalization of positive feelings about self
- ☐ Demonstration of healthy coping strategies
- ☐ Viewing and touching of the incision

Key interventions

- Convey empathy and provide emotional support. Set aside time to discuss the patient's concerns and feelings about body image changes and loss of breast.
- Monitor the patient's behavior, staying alert for mood swings, sadness, tearfulness, and withdrawal from loved ones.
- Encourage the patient to fix her hair, apply makeup, and wear her own nightgowns to help her feel more attractive. Provide affirmation of the patient's femininity to enhance self-confidence.
- Urge the family to support the patient's efforts to adapt to body image changes.
- Evaluate the patient's readiness to look at and touch the incision.
- Encourage the patient to participate in wound care when ready.
- Provide information about breast reconstruction and external breast prosthesis.
- Arrange for the patient to meet others who have adapted to mastectomy successfully.

NURSING DIAGNOSIS

Altered sexuality patterns related to perceived loss of femininity and fear of rejection

DESIRED PATIENT OUTCOME

The patient will express concerns and fears regarding altered sexuality patterns

Outcome measurement criteria

- ☐ Verbalization of feelings regarding loss of breast
- ☐ Discussion of what breast symbolizes to the patient
- ☐ Verbalization of concerns about acceptance or rejection by the partner and family
- ☐ Verbalization of effects of treatment on sexuality
- ☐ Effective communication with partner
- ☐ Verbalization of need for counseling, if applicable

Key interventions

- Provide privacy to discuss the patient's concerns about altered sexuality patterns, perceived loss of femininity, and fear of rejection.
- Maintain nonjudgmental approach.
- Create atmosphere that encourages open expression of feelings. Initiate conversation, such as by saying, "Some women have concerns and fears about their sexuality after a mastectomy. Are there any questions you'd like me to answer?"
- Encourage the patient to discuss concerns with partner. Provide privacy to promote effective communication.
- Maintain positive outlook when discussing sexuality concerns with the patient and partner.

- Counsel the partner to hold and touch the patient, to show love and acceptance. Suggest such activities as cuddling and massage to express intimacy during postoperative period.
- Provide information about local support groups, such as "I Can Cope" and "Reach for Recovery."
- Refer the patient to an appropriate mental health professional for continued counseling after discharge. Stress that recognizing need for counseling indicates strength, not weakness.

NURSING DIAGNOSIS

Knowledge deficit regarding discharge instructions and follow-up care

DESIRED PATIENT OUTCOME

The patient will demonstrate adequate knowledge and skills regarding follow-up care

Outcome measurement criteria

☐ Identification of signs and symptoms of lymphedema

☐ Verbalization of activity limitations

☐ Discussion of techniques to prevent injury

☐ Demonstration of correct exercise techniques

☐ Verbalization of available community resources

☐ Verbalization of importance of follow-up care

Key interventions

- Teach the patient and family about signs and symptoms of lymphedema, such as pain, tightness or tingling, loss of sensation, muscle weakness, or increased circumference of affected arm.

- Explain that acute lymphedema may occur 4 to 6 weeks after surgery and usually is transient, whereas chronic lymphedema may persist for weeks, months, or even years after surgery.
- Advise the patient to report signs and symptoms of lymphedema or infection to the primary health care practitioner immediately.
- Teach wound and drain care techniques. Observe return demonstration.
- Instruct the patient to elevate arm for 30 to 45 minutes every 2 hours for 2 to 3 weeks after discharge, then two to three times daily for 6 weeks.
- Provide the patient with written information on post-discharge exercises, such as wall walking, elbow pull-in, back scratch, and rope pull. Observe return demonstrations to verify correct technique.
- Instruct the patient to avoid carrying luggage, purse, or heavy objects with affected arm.
- Caution the patient to avoid wearing clothing with tight or elastic sleeves.
- Encourage the patient to stop smoking to prevent blood vessel constriction.
- Advise the patient to alert health care providers not to take blood samples or blood pressure measurements in affected arm.
- Inform the patient and family that fatigue is common for up to 6 weeks after surgery and that rest periods are vital to recovery.
- Supply information on radiation or chemotherapy, if applicable.
- Provide written information on available community resources.
- Reinforce importance of follow-up care to monitor progress.

Gynecologic surgery (major)

Surgery involving one or more female reproductive organs, such as oophorectomy (removal of one or both ovaries) or hysterectomy (removal of uterus).

NURSING DIAGNOSIS

Fear related to surgical outcome

DESIRED PATIENT OUTCOME

The patient will express decreased fear about the surgical outcome

Outcome measurement criteria

- ☐ Verbalization of concerns and fears
- ☐ Discussion of surgery and postoperative care
- ☐ Relaxed facial expression and body posture
- ☐ Use of relaxation techniques to decrease fear
- ☐ Verbalization of decreased fear

Key interventions

- Assess anxiety and fear.
- Encourage the patient to express concerns and fears. Determine source of fear, such as fear of cancer diagnosis or loss of reproductive capacity.
- Clarify misconceptions and answer questions honestly.
- Listen for verbal cues that indicate increase or decrease in fear.
- Explain all preoperative and postoperative care.

- Review the patient's role in postoperative care. Stress importance of deep breathing, coughing, early ambulation, and pain control.
- Teach relaxation techniques, such as deep breathing, guided imagery, and music therapy.
- Maintain environment that is conducive to relaxation.

NURSING DIAGNOSIS

Pain related to surgical tissue trauma and manipulation of internal organs

DESIRED PATIENT OUTCOME

The patient will experience relief from pain

Outcome measurement criteria

- ☐ Verbalization of adequate pain relief
- ☐ Vital signs within normal ranges
- ☐ Participation in self-care activities
- ☐ Demonstration of ability to cough, deep-breathe, and ambulate without difficulty
- ☐ Relaxed facial expression and muscle tone
- ☐ Demonstration of correct technique for operating patient-controlled analgesia (PCA) pump, if applicable
- ☐ Demonstration of proper use of pharmacologic and nonpharmacologic pain control measures

Key interventions

- Ask the patient to describe nature, location, and severity of pain.
- Explain principles of pain management, including meaning of *p.r.n.*

- Administer pain medication, as prescribed, before such activities as getting out of bed.
- Evaluate effectiveness of pain medication.
- Encourage the patient to request pain medication before pain becomes severe.
- Discuss use of PCA, if applicable. Teach the patient how to use PCA pump, and observe return demonstration.
- Monitor for respiratory depression and other adverse effects of narcotics, if prescribed.
- Switch to oral analgesics, as ordered, once pain subsides and the patient can tolerate oral intake.
- Reassure the patient and family that postoperative narcotic addiction is unlikely.
- Teach the patient how to use nonpharmacologic pain-control measures.
- Explain that ambulation relieves flatulence.
- Consult the physician or clinical pharmacist if pain management is ineffective.

NURSING DIAGNOSIS

High risk for fluid volume deficit related to surgery

DESIRED PATIENT OUTCOME

The patient will maintain adequate fluid balance

Outcome measurement criteria

- ☐ Balanced fluid intake and output
- ☐ Vital signs within normal ranges
- ☐ Maintenance of hemodynamic stability
- ☐ Urine output of at least 30 ml/hour
- ☐ Normal level of consciousness

- ☐ Hemoglobin and hematocrit values within normal ranges
- ☐ Absence of excessive bleeding from incision
- ☐ Absence of excessive vaginal bleeding

Key interventions

- Assess vital signs frequently after the patient returns from surgery and every 4 hours after her condition stabilizes. Stay alert for signs and symptoms of fluid volume depletion, such as decreasing blood pressure and weak, thready pulse.
- Administer I.V. fluid replacement, as prescribed.
- Measure and document fluid intake and output. Notify the physician if urine output drops below 30 ml/hour.
- Monitor hemoglobin and hematocrit values, and report significant changes to the physician.
- Observe skin color and temperature. Stay alert for signs and symptoms of shock, such as pallor and cool, clammy skin.
- Monitor for changes in level of consciousness.
- Assess surgical dressing frequently for drainage and excessive bleeding. Reinforce dressing, as needed, and notify the physician of significant bleeding.
- Check for excessive vaginal bleeding if vaginal hysterectomy was performed.

NURSING DIAGNOSIS

Ineffective breathing pattern related to incisional pain and narcotic analgesics

DESIRED PATIENT OUTCOME

The patient will maintain an effective breathing pattern

Outcome measurement criteria

- ☐ Respiratory rate of 12 to 20 breaths/minute
- ☐ Absence of adventitious lung sounds
- ☐ Absence of splinting, shallow breathing, and dyspnea
- ☐ Pulse oximetry values within normal range
- ☐ Normal skin color
- ☐ Absence of pneumonia and atelectasis
- ☐ Verbalization of increased breathing comfort
- ☐ Demonstration of correct techniques for coughing, deep breathing, splinting, and using incentive spirometry
- ☐ Demonstration of ability to expectorate secretions

Key interventions

- Assess respiratory status every 4 hours, noting adventitious lung sounds.
- Observe for splinting, shallow breathing, and dyspnea.
- Measure vital signs frequently.
- Monitor pulse oximetry values, and report significant changes to the physician.
- Observe skin for pallor and cyanosis.
- Encourage the patient to turn, cough, and deep-breathe every 2 hours.
- Teach the patient how to splint incision, and observe return demonstration.
- Assist with activities of daily living and ambulation during early postoperative period.

NURSING DIAGNOSIS

High risk for altered peripheral tissue perfusion related to pelvic venous stasis secondary to surgery

DESIRED PATIENT OUTCOME

The patient will maintain adequate peripheral tissue perfusion

Outcome measurement criteria

- ☐ Presence of peripheral pulses
- ☐ Normal skin color and temperature
- ☐ Absence of pain and swelling in thighs and calves
- ☐ Demonstration of ability to perform leg exercises

Key interventions

- Assess for peripheral pulses.
- Evaluate skin color and temperature.
- Ask the patient if she has leg or thigh pain. Encourage her to report such pain promptly.
- Apply antiembolism stockings, as ordered. Remove stockings for 1 hour each shift and reapply.
- Avoid placing pillows under the patient's knees or raising knee gatch on bed because doing so may impede leg circulation.
- Avoid placing the patient in high Fowler's position, which impedes pelvic venous return.
- Place bed in flat position for short intervals every 2 hours to promote venous return.
- Teach correct technique for leg exercises. Encourage the patient to perform exercises every hour while she's awake until she begins ambulating.
- Encourage and assist the patient with early ambulation. Stay alert for signs and symptoms of orthostatic hypotension, such as weakness, dizziness, and fainting.

Nursing Diagnosis

High risk for infection related to surgical tissue trauma

DESIRED PATIENT OUTCOME

The patient will remain free of infection

Outcome measurement criteria

- ☐ Oral temperature at or below 99.0° F (37.2° C)
- ☐ White blood cell (WBC) count within normal range
- ☐ Absence of erythema, purulent drainage, and tenderness at incision site
- ☐ Negative blood and wound cultures

Key interventions

- Measure oral temperature at least every 4 hours.
- Observe for chills, fever, diaphoresis, and changes in vital signs.
- Monitor WBC count, and report significant increases to the physician.
- Assess wound each shift for signs of infection, such as warmth, redness, drainage, tenderness, and odor.
- Obtain blood and wound cultures, as needed and ordered, and monitor results.
- Consult the infection control practitioner, as needed.

Nursing Diagnosis

High risk for urinary retention related to surgical bladder manipulation

DESIRED PATIENT OUTCOME

The patient will maintain adequate fluid output

Outcome measurement criteria

- ☐ Urine output of at least 30 ml/hour
- ☐ Balanced fluid intake and output
- ☐ Absence of signs and symptoms of bladder distention
- ☐ Normal urine color
- ☐ Verbalization of increased comfort

Key interventions

- Assess frequently for signs and symptoms of bladder distention, such as restlessness, pain, and urinary urgency.
- Measure and document fluid intake and output. Be aware that urine output should be at least 30 ml/hour. Notify the physician if fluid intake exceeds output.
- Observe for increased restlessness and discomfort. Encourage the patient to report bladder discomfort promptly.
- If urinary catheter is present, maintain patency of catheter and drainage tubing.
- Once catheter is removed, observe the patient's ability to void. Use interventions to stimulate voiding, such as running tap water or pouring warm water over abdomen.
- Monitor for signs and symptoms of urinary retention, such as reduced urine flow and distended bladder. Catheterize the patient, if ordered, to measure residual urine.
- Assist the patient to void on commode rather than in bedpan to promote complete bladder emptying.

NURSING DIAGNOSIS

Constipation related to decreased gastric motility secondary to narcotics and reduced oral intake

DESIRED PATIENT OUTCOME

The patient will regain normal bowel function

Outcome measurement criteria

- ☐ Presence of bowel sounds
- ☐ Resumption of bowel movements
- ☐ Absence of abdominal distention
- ☐ Absence of constipation
- ☐ Adequate fluid intake

Key interventions

- Assess abdomen every 4 hours. Listen for bowel sounds in all quadrants.
- Observe for abdominal distention and tension on suture line.
- Monitor for first postoperative bowel movement.
- Evaluate color, consistency, frequency, and amount of stools.
- Notify the physician if bowel sounds do not resume or if bowel movement does not occur by specified time.
- Offer fluids and increased dietary fiber to promote normal bowel function.
- Evaluate dietary intake, and advance diet, as tolerated.
- Encourage early ambulation to decrease flatulence.

NURSING DIAGNOSIS

Anticipatory grieving related to loss of reproductive capacity or possible cancer diagnosis

DESIRED PATIENT OUTCOME

The patient will exhibit positive coping mechanisms to deal with grief

Outcome measurement criteria

- ☐ Identification of perceived loss
- ☐ Verbalization of feelings about loss
- ☐ Verbalization of understanding of grief process
- ☐ Use of healthy coping mechanisms to deal with perceived loss
- ☐ Participation in care and treatment decisions
- ☐ Participation in self-care activities
- ☐ Identification of appropriate support systems
- ☐ Demonstration of willingness to accept support from others
- ☐ Verbalization of need for counseling, if applicable

Key interventions

- Encourage the patient to discuss concerns and fears.
- Help the patient identify perceived loss. Be aware that a woman of childbearing age, whether childless or not, may have intense feelings of loss over inability to reproduce. She also may be struggling with potential cancer diagnosis.
- Encourage the patient and family to express feelings about perceived loss and its effects on their well-being and lifestyle.
- Assist the patient and family to understand grief process. Explain that feelings of grief and loss are normal in such circumstances.
- Help the patient identify strengths and strategies she has used successfully to cope with difficult situations in past. Encourage her to adapt these strategies to current situation and to draw on others' strength to enhance her coping ability.
- Allow the patient to participate in care and treatment decisions.

- Encourage the patient to participate in self-care activities, as tolerated. Offer positive reinforcement for participation.
- Help the patient identify support systems, such as family, friends, and clergy. Encourage her to accept their help.
- Provide the patient and family with information about community support groups and programs.
- Discuss possible need for counseling after discharge. Refer the patient to a mental health professional, if appropriate.

NURSING DIAGNOSIS

High risk for altered sexuality patterns related to perceived change in body image secondary to surgery

DESIRED PATIENT OUTCOME

The patient will discuss concerns about sexuality

Outcome measurement criteria

- ☐ Verbalization of feelings about actual or perceived changes in sexuality patterns
- ☐ Verbalization of feelings about body image and self-concept
- ☐ Demonstration of interest in personal appearance
- ☐ Discussion of effects of surgery on sexuality
- ☐ Demonstration of effective communication with partner
- ☐ Verbalization of need for counseling, if applicable

Key interventions

- Provide privacy to discuss the patient's concerns about actual or perceived sexuality changes.

- Encourage the patient to express feelings about body image and self-concept. Offer validation and acceptance of her feelings.
- Maintain nonjudgmental approach. Create atmosphere that encourages open expression of feelings.
- Provide the patient and partner with information about her condition and its treatment. Answer questions and clarify misconceptions.
- Encourage the patient to discuss concerns with partner. Provide privacy to promote effective communication.
- Explain that altered hormone levels may cause such transient changes as vaginal dryness, decreased vaginal sensitivity, and reduced libido.
- Suggest such activities as holding hands, cuddling, and giving massages to express intimacy during postoperative period.
- Advise the patient to avoid scxual intercourse for 4 to 6 weeks. Mention that return to full sexual function may take up to 4 months.
- Discuss ways to prevent discomfort and conserve energy once intercourse resumes, such as using water-based vaginal lubricant, avoiding positions that place pressure on incision, and having intercourse when the patient's energy level is high.
- Encourage the patient to participate in activities associated with femininity, such as fixing her hair, applying makeup, and wearing her own clothes rather than hospital gown.
- Provide information about local support groups, such as "I Can Cope," for patients with cancer.
- Offer referral to an appropriate mental health professional or sex counselor. Stress that recognizing need for counseling is sign of strength, not weakness.

NURSING DIAGNOSIS

Knowledge deficit regarding follow-up care

DESIRED PATIENT OUTCOME

The patient will express an understanding of required follow-up care

Outcome measurement criteria

- ☐ Verbalization of activity restrictions
- ☐ Identification of signs and symptoms of infection and thrombophlebitis
- ☐ Demonstration of correct wound care technique, if applicable
- ☐ Verbalization of prescribed medication regimen
- ☐ Verbalization of understanding of hormone replacement therapy, if prescribed
- ☐ Verbalization of need to keep follow-up gynecologic appointments
- ☐ Verbalization of understanding of usual course of recovery

Key interventions

- Review nature of surgery and its consequences. Explain that the patient no longer will have menstrual periods and will be unable to become pregnant.
- Clarify misconceptions about sequelae of hysterectomy, if applicable, including facial hair development, masculine appearance, marked weight gain, depression, and nervousness.
- Teach correct wound care technique, and observe return demonstration.
- Teach the patient how to care for indwelling urinary (Foley) catheter, if applicable.

- Review names, purposes, dosages, and common adverse effects of prescribed drugs.
- Instruct the patient to report fever, incisional tenderness, and excessive or odorous drainage.
- Teach the patient to observe vaginal discharge daily. Explain that small spots of blood and brownish stains are normal and may last for up to 1 week. Emphasize importance of notifying the primary health care practitioner of menstrual-like bleeding, severe cramps, and hot flashes.
- Advise the patient to immediately report signs and symptoms of thrombophlebitis, such as leg or thigh pain or swelling.
- Encourage the patient to walk or perform similar activity daily.
- Caution the patient not to perform strenuous activity or lift objects over 20 lb (9 kg) for 6 weeks.
- Explain that the patient can resume driving in 3 to 4 weeks.
- Advise the patient not to use tampons or douches for 6 weeks or until approved by the physician.
- If the patient has had both ovaries removed, advise her to report menopausal signs and symptoms and see the physician every 6 months to evaluate effectiveness of hormone replacement therapy, if prescribed.
- Inform the patient that although depression commonly follows gynecologic surgery, she should seek help if she thinks that she cannot function normally.

Penile prosthesis implantation

Insertion of semirigid or inflatable device in penis to restore erectile function.

NURSING DIAGNOSIS

Fear related to surgery and uncertain outcome

DESIRED PATIENT OUTCOME

The patient will express decreased fear about surgery and its outcome

Outcome measurement criteria

☐ Verbalization of concerns and fears

☐ Discussion of surgery and postoperative care

☐ Relaxed facial expression and posture

☐ Use of relaxation techniques to control fear

☐ Verbalization of decreased fear

Key interventions

- Assess for anxiety and fear.
- Encourage the patient to express concerns and fears.
- Determine source of fear. Clarify misconceptions and answer questions honestly.
- Listen for verbal cues that indicate increased fear.
- Acknowledge that the patient may be embarrassed by nature of surgery.
- Explain all preoperative and postoperative care.
- Review the patient's expected role in postoperative care.

- Teach relaxation techniques, such as deep breathing, meditation, guided imagery, and music therapy.
- Maintain environment that is conducive to relaxation.

NURSING DIAGNOSIS

High risk for infection related to implantation of prosthetic device

DESIRED PATIENT OUTCOME

The patient will remain free of infection

Outcome measurement criteria

- ☐ Oral temperature at or below 99.0° F (37.2° C)
- ☐ White blood cell (WBC) count within normal range
- ☐ Absence of redness, warmth, tenderness, and odorous drainage at incision site

Key interventions

- Measure oral temperature every 4 hours after immediate postoperative period.
- Monitor WBC count, and report significant increases to the physician.
- Assess wound for signs and symptoms of infection, such as redness, warmth, tenderness, and odorous drainage.
- Administer antibiotics, as prescribed, to ensure therapeutic blood levels.

NURSING DIAGNOSIS

Pain related to surgical trauma

DESIRED PATIENT OUTCOME

The patient will experience relief from pain

Outcome measurement criteria

- ☐ Verbalization of adequate pain relief
- ☐ Vital signs within normal ranges
- ☐ Relaxed facial expression and muscle tone
- ☐ Participation in self-care activities
- ☐ Demonstration of use of pharmacologic and comfort measures

Key interventions

- Ask the patient to describe nature, location, and severity of pain.
- Explain principles of postoperative pain management, including meaning of *p.r.n.*
- Reassure the patient that scrotal pain is temporary and that scrotal bruising and swelling will subside after about 2 weeks.
- Advise the patient to wear comfortable knit undershorts to minimize movement of penis and scrotum and to increase comfort.
- Administer pain medication, as prescribed, before such activities as getting out of bed.
- Encourage the patient to request pain medication before pain becomes severe.
- Switch to oral analgesics, as ordered, when pain decreases.
- Evaluate effectiveness of pain management.
- Consult the physician or clinical pharmacist if pain management is ineffective.

NURSING DIAGNOSIS

Situational low self-esteem related to sexual dysfunction

DESIRED PATIENT OUTCOME

The patient will express positive feelings about himself

Outcome measurement criteria

- ☐ Verbalization of feelings about medical condition and its effect on self-esteem
- ☐ Participation in self-care activities
- ☐ Participation in care and treatment decisions
- ☐ Verbalization of sense of control over life events
- ☐ Verbalization of positive feelings about self

Key interventions

- Provide uninterrupted time to discuss the patient's concerns.
- Encourage the patient to express feelings about need for penile prosthesis and its impact on self-esteem.
- Provide reassurance about prosthesis and its effect on erectile function.
- Help the patient to identify strengths and recognize that self-worth does not hinge on sexual ability.
- Maintain open, nonjudgmental attitude.
- Allow the patient to participate in care and treatment decisions.
- Encourage participation in self-care activities.
- Provide positive reinforcement for behavior or statements that indicate that the patient is regaining positive feelings about himself.
- Encourage the patient to seek counseling if concerns about sexuality and self-esteem cause ongoing distress.
- Provide information about local support groups and counseling services.

NURSING DIAGNOSIS

Knowledge deficit regarding follow-up care

DESIRED PATIENT OUTCOME

The patient will express an understanding of required follow-up care

Outcome measurement criteria

- ☐ Verbalization of activity restrictions
- ☐ Identification of signs and symptoms of infection
- ☐ Identification of signs and symptoms of erosion of prosthetic device
- ☐ Demonstration of correct wound care technique
- ☐ Demonstration of correct technique for inflating and deflating an inflatable prosthesis

Key interventions

- Demonstrate correct technique for inflating and deflating an inflatable prosthesis to the patient and his partner. Stress importance of inflating and deflating prosthesis repeatedly before initial use to build up fibrous sheath around device.
- Advise the patient to avoid contact sports, heavy lifting, and sexual activity for 3 weeks after surgery.
- Teach the patient to report signs and symptoms of infection at the incision site, such as fever, redness, warmth, swelling, and drainage.
- Instruct the patient to report signs and symptoms of erosion of prosthetic device, such as pallor and thinning of skin near glans penis and changes in size, color, or contour of penis.
- Discuss ways to conceal semirigid prosthetic device with clothing.

Prostate cancer

Cancerous tumor that arises from parenchymal cells of prostate gland.

NURSING DIAGNOSIS

Pain related to cancer metastasis to vertebra or spine

DESIRED PATIENT OUTCOME

The patient will experience relief from pain

Outcome measurement criteria

☐ Verbalization of adequate pain relief

☐ Vital signs within normal ranges

☐ Relaxed facial expression and muscle tone

☐ Demonstration of ability to self-administer prescribed medication, if applicable

Key interventions

- Assess for signs and symptoms of pain, such as increased blood pressure, facial grimacing, shallow breathing, restlessness, and irritability. Be aware that prostate cancer may cause pain in lower back, pelvis, or upper thighs.
- Encourage the patient to request pain medication before pain becomes severe.
- Discuss pain control with the patient, family, and physician to help develop pain management plan.
- Recommend use of patient-controlled analgesia (PCA), if applicable, to provide increased control over pain management. Teach the patient and family how to use PCA pump, and observe return demonstrations.

- If the patient becomes unable to operate PCA pump because of diminished level of consciousness, ask the physician to consider continuous analgesic infusion for maximal comfort.
- Change the patient's position slowly to avoid injury.
- Provide physical support when the patient moves in bed or ambulates to promote comfort and prevent injury.
- Place the patient in whirlpool bath or apply heat to relax muscles and reduce pain.
- Offer massage to relax muscles.
- Mention that the patient may receive corticosteroids to counteract bone pain.
- Discuss possible use of hormone therapy in treating metastatic prostate cancer.
- Monitor and document effectiveness of pain management.
- Consult the physician and clinical pharmacist if pain management is ineffective.

NURSING DIAGNOSIS

Fear related to complex treatment options, altered sexuality, and prognosis

DESIRED PATIENT OUTCOME

The patient will express decreased fear

Outcome measurement criteria

- ☐ Verbalization of concerns and fears
- ☐ Discussion of treatment options and related care
- ☐ Relaxed facial expression and posture
- ☐ Use of relaxation techniques to control fear
- ☐ Verbalization of decreased fear

☐ Participation in care and treatment decisions

☐ Participation in self-care activities, as tolerated

Key interventions

- Assess for anxiety and fear.
- Listen for verbal cues that indicate increased fear.
- Determine source of fear. Clarify misconceptions and answer questions honestly.
- Encourage the patient to express concerns about treatment options, altered sexuality, and prognosis.
- Teach relaxation techniques, such as deep breathing, guided imagery, and music therapy.
- Maintain environment that is conducive to relaxation.
- Discuss alternate ways to express sexuality. Explain value of sexual counseling, and mention possibility of recovering some or all sexual function after treatment ends.
- Help the patient identify skills used to solve problems in past. Assist the patient in adapting these skills to current situation.
- Allow the patient to participate in care and treatment decisions.
- Encourage participation in self-care activities, as tolerated.
- Contact the patient's clergyperson or the hospital chaplain, if appropriate.

NURSING DIAGNOSIS

Altered urinary elimination related to obstruction of urethra by enlarged prostate gland

DESIRED PATIENT OUTCOME

The patient will achieve maximal urinary elimination within physiologic limitations

Outcome measurement criteria

- ☐ Adequate urine output
- ☐ Balanced fluid intake and output
- ☐ Demonstration of ability to start and stop urine stream
- ☐ Absence of urinary urgency, frequency, and dysuria
- ☐ Absence of bladder distention
- ☐ Absence of signs and symptoms of fluid retention
- ☐ Blood urea nitrogen (BUN) and serum creatinine levels within normal ranges
- ☐ Urine specific gravity within normal range

Key interventions

- Measure and document fluid intake and output each shift. Notify the physician if output drops below 30 ml/hour or if intake exceeds output.
- Ask the patient if he has difficulty starting or stopping urine stream.
- Assess for bladder distention (a sign of urine retention) every shift.
- Stress importance of promptly reporting signs and symptoms of urinary obstruction or infection, such as urinary frequency and urgency and dysuria.
- Monitor BUN and serum creatinine levels and urine specific gravity for evidence of decreased renal function.
- Observe for edema and weight gain, which may indicate fluid retention.
- Perform urinary catheterization only if needed to relieve urinary retention.

NURSING DIAGNOSIS

Altered protection related to immunosuppression secondary to chemotherapy or radiation therapy

DESIRED PATIENT OUTCOME

The patient will remain free of infection

Outcome measurement criteria

- ☐ Oral temperature at or below 99.0° F (37.2° C)
- ☐ White blood cell (WBC) count within expected range
- ☐ Negative blood cultures

Key interventions

- Measure oral temperature at least every 8 hours, and report elevations to the physician.
- Monitor WBC count, and report significant increases to the physician.
- Monitor blood culture results, as indicated.
- Wash hands diligently to prevent cross-contamination.
- Maintain strict asepsis during invasive procedures.
- Consult the infection control practitioner, if needed.

NURSING DIAGNOSIS

Altered nutrition: less than body requirements related to nausea, vomiting, and anorexia secondary to chemotherapy

DESIRED PATIENT OUTCOME

The patient will increase nutritional intake

Outcome measurement criteria

- ☐ Maintenance of or increase in weight

- ☐ Demonstration of adequate caloric intake
- ☐ Participation in food selection
- ☐ Serum albumin and protein levels within normal ranges
- ☐ Absence of severe nausea and vomiting
- ☐ Absence of oral mucous membrane lesions
- ☐ Identification of measures that help control nausea and vomiting
- ☐ Verbalization of need to report significant weight loss to the primary health care practitioner

Key interventions

- Obtain baseline weight on admission, and weigh daily to determine progress and detect fluid retention.
- Assess bowel sounds each shift.
- Monitor serum albumin and protein levels to assess nutritional status.
- Administer antiemetics before chemotherapy, as prescribed.
- Assess oral cavity and mucous membranes for stomatitis.
- Allow the patient to rest before meals.
- Discuss food preferences, and encourage the patient to participate in food selection.
- Provide oral hygiene before meals, using mild mouthwash and viscous Xylocaine.
- Serve small, frequent meals of nutritious soft foods and fluids.
- Ask the family to bring the patient's favorite foods from home within dietary restrictions.
- Encourage the family to visit during meals to enhance the patient's meal enjoyment.
- Consult the dietitian for appropriate calorie count and nutritional assessment, if needed.

Prostatectomy

Partial or complete surgical removal of prostate gland.

NURSING DIAGNOSIS

High risk for fluid volume deficit related to postoperative bleeding

DESIRED PATIENT OUTCOME

The patient will maintain adequate fluid balance

Outcome measurement criteria

- ☐ Balanced fluid intake and output
- ☐ Vital signs within normal ranges
- ☐ Absence of excessive bleeding from incision
- ☐ Absence of clots, bright red blood, and persistent burgundy-colored blood from urinary catheter
- ☐ Hemoglobin and hematocrit values within normal ranges
- ☐ Normal level of consciousness

Key interventions

- Assess vital signs frequently during immediate postoperative period and then every 4 hours once the patient becomes stable. Stay alert for signs and symptoms of fluid volume depletion, such as decreasing blood pressure and weak, thready pulse.
- Observe skin color and temperature. Stay alert for signs and symptoms of shock, such as pallor and cool, clammy skin.
- Monitor for changes in level of consciousness.

- Encourage fluid intake of 3,000 ml/day, unless contraindicated.
- Administer I.V. fluids, as prescribed.
- Measure and document fluid intake and output.
- Monitor hemoglobin and hematocrit values, and report significant changes to the physician.
- Assess surgical dressing for drainage or excessive bleeding every hour for first 12 to 24 hours. Reinforce dressing, as needed, and notify the physician of abnormal bleeding.
- Maintain continuous bladder irrigation, as ordered, to prevent clot formation.
- Maintain traction on urinary catheter for 6 to 8 hours, as ordered.
- Measure and document amount of bleeding and presence of clots in urinary drainage. Notify the surgeon of bright red blood, persistent burgundy-colored blood, or persistent clot formation in drainage.
- Avoid placing the patient upright because this may increase pressure on incision and heighten risk of bleeding.
- Administer stool softeners and laxatives, as ordered, to prevent constipation and reduce risk of bleeding and rectal tears. Advise the patient to consume more dietary fiber and drink prune juice.
- Caution the patient not to strain during bowel movements because this may cause bleeding, especially if the surgeon used retropubic or perineal approach.
- Avoid use of rectal thermometers, rectal tubes, and enemas for at least 1 week.

NURSING DIAGNOSIS

High risk for infection related to surgical trauma

DESIRED PATIENT OUTCOME

The patient will remain free of infection

Outcome measurement criteria

- ☐ Oral temperature at or below 99.0° F (37.2° C)
- ☐ White blood cell (WBC) count within normal range
- ☐ Absence of erythema, purulent drainage, and tenderness at incision site
- ☐ Clear urine
- ☐ Negative blood cultures

Key interventions

- Measure oral temperature at least every 4 hours.
- Observe for chills, fever, diaphoresis, and changes in vital signs.
- Monitor WBC count, and report significant increases to the physician.
- Assess wound each shift for warmth, redness, drainage, tenderness, and odor.
- Perform meticulous catheter care daily.
- Maintain catheter patency to prevent clotting and urinary stasis, which may lead to infection.
- Encourage adequate fluid intake to maintain urine output of at least 1,500 ml/day and flush bacteria from urinary tract.
- Send urine samples for culture and sensitivity testing, as ordered. Report significant findings to the physician.
- Consult the infection control practitioner, as needed.

NURSING DIAGNOSIS

Pain related to bladder spasms, urinary retention, and surgical trauma

DESIRED PATIENT OUTCOME

The patient will experience relief from pain

Outcome measurement criteria

- ☐ Verbalization of adequate pain relief
- ☐ Vital signs within normal ranges
- ☐ Absence of bladder distention and spasms
- ☐ Absence of urine leakage around catheter

Key interventions

- Assess for signs and symptoms of pain, such as increased blood pressure, shallow breathing, facial grimacing, restlessness, and irritability.
- Administer analgesics and antispasmodic drugs, as prescribed.
- Encourage the patient to request pain medication before pain becomes severe.
- Provide alternative pain-relief measures, such as heat application to rectum or sitz baths if the patient underwent perineal prostatectomy.
- Evaluate and document effectiveness of pain management.
- Observe catheter tubing for kinks and other obstructions.
- Check for bladder distention.
- Stay alert for complaints that may indicate bladder spasm, such as sharp, intermittent pain; urinary urgency; and urine leakage around catheter.
- Explain that bladder spasms will become milder and less frequent within 24 to 48 hours.
- Irrigate catheter, as ordered, to relieve obstruction.

- Mention that catheter will cause sensation of fullness and that straining to pass urine around it will cause bladder spasms.

NURSING DIAGNOSIS

Urge incontinence related to catheter removal and changes in sphincter tone

DESIRED PATIENT OUTCOME

The patient will regain control of urination

Outcome measurement criteria

☐ Resumption of normal voiding pattern

☐ Absence of incontinence

☐ Absence of postvoiding residual volume

☐ Clean, dry perineal region

Key interventions

- Assess for urinary dribbling after catheter removal.
- Measure residual urine volume through suprapubic tube, if applicable. Notify the physician if volume exceeds 50 ml.
- Observe and document voiding pattern, noting time and amount of each voiding.
- Instruct the patient to void no more than once every 2 hours during first 24 hours after surgery.
- Explain that urine may leak around incision site initially, depending on surgical approach.
- Reassure the patient that some incontinence is expected after catheter removal because of weakened sphincter.
- Teach the patient to strengthen his sphincter by tightening buttocks for 5 to 10 seconds 10 to 20 times per hour.

- Explain that although normal urinary control usually returns within 2 to 3 weeks after most prostate procedures, it may take up to 6 months after perineal prostatectomy.
- Encourage the patient to use disposable incontinence pads to promote comfort.

NURSING DIAGNOSIS

High risk for sexual dysfunction related to surgery

DESIRED PATIENT OUTCOME

The patient will adapt to changes in sexual function

Outcome measurement criteria

- ☐ Verbalization of potential sexual dysfunction
- ☐ Verbalization of concerns and fears about sexual dysfunction
- ☐ Description of relation between illness and sexual dysfunction
- ☐ Effective communication of concerns with partner
- ☐ Demonstration of willingness to obtain counseling, if appropriate

Key interventions

- Provide environment in which the patient is comfortable discussing sexuality concerns.
- Discuss expected effects of prostatectomy on sexual function. Include the partner in discussion to promote communication.

- Explain that retrograde ejaculation is common after transurethral retrograde prostatectomy and suprapubic prostatectomy. Mention that this condition will not interfere with sexual activity, although it does cause sterility. Reassure the patient that normal ejaculation will return within several months.
- Mention that radical prostatectomy severs perineal nerves and, therefore, usually causes impotence.
- Urge the patient to discuss with the physician the possibility of receiving penile implant.
- Inform the patient who has erectile capability that he may resume intercourse in 4 to 6 weeks.
- Urge the patient to share his feelings with his partner.
- Explain to the partner that feelings of loss, grief, anger, and fear are common in patients who have had prostatectomy.
- Refer the patient and partner to appropriate support groups and counselors.

NURSING DIAGNOSIS

Knowledge deficit regarding follow-up care

DESIRED PATIENT OUTCOME

The patient will exhibit adequate understanding and skills to complete his recovery at home

Outcome measurement criteria

- ☐ Verbalization of physical and sexual activity limitations
- ☐ Description of medication regimen
- ☐ Demonstration of correct wound care technique
- ☐ Demonstration of correct drainage tube or catheter care technique
- ☐ Verbalization of need for follow-up evaluation

Key interventions

- Teach the patient and family correct wound care technique. Observe return demonstrations.
- Instruct the patient and family in proper catheter or drainage tube care, if applicable. Observe return demonstrations.
- Review names, purposes, dosages, and common adverse effects of prescribed drugs. Provide supplemental written information for use as reference.
- If the patient will be discharged on antibiotics, stress the need to complete entire course of medication to prevent infection.
- Encourage the patient to avoid sitting upright until incision heals to decrease risk of bleeding.
- Advise the patient to avoid straining during bowel movements for 4 to 6 weeks. Encourage increased fluid intake and use of stool softeners and laxatives to maintain normal bowel activity.
- Inform the patient that he may resume sexual activity in 4 to 6 weeks.
- Advise the patient to report incisional bleeding and signs or symptoms of infection to the primary health care practitioner immediately.
- Teach the patient to avoid heavy lifting and strenuous activity for 4 to 6 weeks.
- Emphasize need for continued follow-up care to monitor progress.

Testicular cancer

Cancer of testicle characterized by small, hard, painless lump in testicle, heavy sensation in testicle, fluid accumulation in scrotum, and perineal pain; most common type of cancer in men aged 15 to 35.

NURSING DIAGNOSIS

Fear related to possible infertility and death secondary to cancer diagnosis

DESIRED PATIENT OUTCOME

The patient will express decreased fear

Outcome measurement criteria

- ☐ Verbalization of concerns and fears
- ☐ Verbalization of decreased fear
- ☐ Relaxed facial expression and posture
- ☐ Use of relaxation techniques to control fear
- ☐ Discussion of care and treatment options
- ☐ Participation in care and treatment decisions
- ☐ Participation in self-care activities, as tolerated

Key interventions

- Assess the patient for anxiety and fear.
- Determine source of fear. Clarify any misconceptions and answer questions honestly.
- Encourage the patient to express concerns and fears about sexuality changes, treatment options, and prognosis.

- Listen for verbal cues that indicate increased fear.
- Allow time for denial, a normal response to diagnosis of testicular cancer.
- Help the patient identify strategies he has used successfully to cope with difficult situations in past. Help him adapt these strategies to current situation.
- Reassure the patient that testicular cancer responds well to radiation therapy if detected early and that it has cure rate of up to 90%. Explain that external beam radiation is directed at abdominal area after testicle removal and that normal testicle is shielded but receives scattered radiation.
- Allow the patient to participate in care and treatment decisions.
- Encourage participation in self-care activities, as tolerated.
- Teach the patient relaxation techniques, such as deep breathing, guided imagery, and music therapy.
- Maintain environment that is conducive to relaxation.
- Ask the physician to discuss effects of cancer on the patient's fertility.
- Provide information on sperm banking and sexuality counseling, if appropriate.
- Contact the patient's clergyperson or the hospital chaplain, if appropriate.

NURSING DIAGNOSIS

Body image disturbance related to scrotal changes and possible breast enlargement

DESIRED PATIENT OUTCOME

The patient will adapt to changes in body image

Outcome measurement criteria

- ☐ Identification of body image changes
- ☐ Verbalization of feelings about body image changes
- ☐ Verbalization of positive feelings about self
- ☐ Demonstration of healthy coping mechanisms
- ☐ Demonstration of willingness to look at and touch scrotum

Key interventions

- Encourage the patient to discuss concerns and feelings about body image changes and their impact on self-concept.
- Validate the patient's feelings and reassure him that he can overcome current crisis.
- Explore the patient's feelings about effects of body image changes on his appearance.
- Help the patient identify strategies he has used successfully to cope with difficult situations in past. Help him adapt these strategies to current situation.
- Provide positive reinforcement for the patient's efforts to use healthy coping mechanisms.
- Discuss ability of healthy testicle to compensate for lack of function in other testicle and thereby minimize changes in male characteristics.
- Explain that breast enlargement is rare but may occur with more advanced forms of testicular cancer.
- Provide information about testicular implant, which can be inserted during initial surgery to minimize disfigurement. Encourage the patient to discuss this option with the physician.
- Involve the patient in self-care activities. When appropriate, encourage him to look at and touch scrotum.

- Teach the patient how to perform testicular self-examination, and observe return demonstration. Provide written material for use as reference.

NURSING DIAGNOSIS

Pain related to pressure from tumor or metastases to groin, retroperitoneal nodes, chest, or abdomen

DESIRED PATIENT OUTCOME

The patient will express relief from pain

Outcome measurement criteria

- ☐ Verbalization of adequate pain control
- ☐ Vital signs within normal ranges
- ☐ Relaxed facial expression and muscle tone
- ☐ Demonstration of use of heat therapy to ease pain

Key interventions

- Assess for signs and symptoms of pain, such as increased blood pressure, facial grimacing, shallow breathing, restlessness, and irritability.
- Encourage the patient to request pain medication before pain becomes severe.
- Provide alternative pain-relief measures, such as massage and use of scrotal support.
- Handle scrotal area gently during examination to decrease discomfort.
- Use heating pad, hot water bottle, warm compresses, or warm bath water to promote circulation and decrease edema.
- Teach relaxation techniques, such as deep breathing, meditation, and guided imagery.

- Monitor and document effectiveness of pain management.
- Consult the physician and clinical pharmacist if pain management is ineffective.

NURSING DIAGNOSIS

Knowledge deficit regarding postoperative care

DESIRED PATIENT OUTCOME

The patient will express an understanding of postoperative care

Outcome measurement criteria

- ☐ Identification of common postoperative complications
- ☐ Verbalization of activity restrictions
- ☐ Demonstration of correct technique for testicular self-examination

Key interventions

- Explain that edema and intrascrotal hemorrhage are most common postoperative complications.
- Place rubber glove filled with crushed ice on scrotum for first 12 hours to control postoperative edema.
- Explain that scrotum will be covered with compression dressing for 3 to 5 days to control intrascrotal bleeding.
- Instruct the patient to report increasing discomfort immediately.
- Teach the patient to avoid prolonged standing, which increases edema.
- Encourage the patient to wear athletic supporter or tight undershorts until healing is complete.
- Caution the patient to avoid heavy lifting for 4 to 6 weeks.

- Encourage the patient to take 20-minute baths three times daily for 1 week after discharge to promote healing and comfort.
- Teach the patient how to perform testicular self-examination, and observe return demonstration. Provide written material for use as reference.
- Stress lifelong need for routine medical evaluations.

Amputation

Surgical removal of part or all of an extremity, performed to remove cancerous tumor or to treat severe trauma, advanced atherosclerosis, or gangrene.

NURSING DIAGNOSIS

High risk for fluid volume deficit related to postoperative hemorrhage

DESIRED PATIENT OUTCOME

The patient will maintain an adequate fluid balance

Outcome measurement criteria

- ☐ Vital signs within normal ranges
- ☐ Balanced fluid intake and output
- ☐ Hemoglobin and hematocrit values within normal ranges
- ☐ Absence of signs or symptoms of active hemorrhage
- ☐ Absence of excessive drainage from surgical site

Key interventions

- Monitor vital signs at least every 4 hours after immediate postoperative period. Stay alert for decreasing blood pressure and weak, thready pulse, which may indicate shock.
- Record fluid intake and output.
- Provide fluid replacement therapy, as ordered.

- Monitor hemoglobin and hematocrit values, and report significant changes to the physician.
- Assess surgical dressing frequently for excessive bloody drainage. Expect minimal oozing. Report significant bleeding to the physician immediately.
- Monitor drainage device for increased amounts of bright red drainage.
- Maintain pressure dressing on stump, as ordered. Reinforce dressing, as needed, but do not change surgical dressing unless ordered by the physician.
- If hemorrhage occurs, apply direct pressure to site to control bleeding. Stay with the patient and notify the physician immediately.

NURSING DIAGNOSIS

High risk for infection related to effects of disruption in skin integrity and preexisting medical condition

DESIRED PATIENT OUTCOME

The patient will remain free of infection

Outcome measurement criteria

- ☐ Oral temperature at or below 99.0° F (37.2° C)
- ☐ White blood cell (WBC) count within normal range
- ☐ Absence of redness, swelling, warmth, and purulent drainage at incision site
- ☐ Demonstration of correct stump care technique
- ☐ Verbalization of signs and symptoms of stump breakdown
- ☐ Demonstration of skin-toughening exercises

Key interventions

- Measure temperature at least every 4 hours after immediate postoperative period. Observe for chills, flushing, and diaphoresis.
- Monitor WBC count, and report significant changes to the physician.
- Observe incision for redness, swelling, warmth, odor, and purulent drainage with each dressing change.
- Use sterile technique during dressing changes. Rewrap stump securely but not tightly.
- Bathe stump daily with mild soap and water, once dressing is no longer needed. Dry stump thoroughly and expose it to air for 20 minutes twice daily.
- If the patient is incontinent, cover stump with plastic to prevent contamination.
- Teach the patient and family correct stump care technique. Observe return demonstration.
- Instruct the patient and family to observe stump daily for signs of breakdown, such as edema, redness, and skin breaks.
- Teach skin-toughening exercises to prepare the patient for prosthesis and reduce risk of infection from skin breakdown. Instruct the patient to press stump against soft pillow four to six times a day, gradually increasing resistance.

NURSING DIAGNOSIS

Pain related to effects of tissue, nerve, and bone trauma

DESIRED PATIENT OUTCOME

The patient will verbalize relief from pain

Outcome measurement criteria

- ☐ Verbalization of adequate pain relief
- ☐ Relaxed facial expression and muscle tone
- ☐ Vital signs within normal ranges
- ☐ Verbalization of understanding of phantom limb pain phenomenon
- ☐ Demonstration of correct use of patient-controlled analgesia (PCA) pump, if applicable

Key interventions

- Assess for nonverbal signs of pain, such as increased blood pressure, facial grimaces, shallow breathing, and restlessness.
- Explain principles of pain management, including meaning of *p.r.n.*
- Encourage the patient to request pain medication before pain becomes severe.
- Use additional pain control methods, such as relaxation, music therapy, guided imagery, and back rubs as an adjunct to analgesics.
- Teach the patient correct use of PCA pump, if ordered. Observe return demonstration.
- Gently massage stump every 4 hours after dressing has been removed. Do not use emollients because these may cause skin maceration.
- Reposition the patient every 2 to 3 hours to relieve discomfort.
- Explain that pain will diminish within 3 to 4 days after surgery.
- Discuss phantom limb pain phenomenon with the patient and family. Explain that this phenomenon is normal response to amputation and may last up to 6 months after surgery.

NURSING DIAGNOSIS

Impaired physical mobility related to weakness

DESIRED PATIENT OUTCOME

The patient will regain mobility after wound healing

Outcome measurement criteria

- ☐ Absence of edema and joint contracture
- ☐ Demonstration of range-of-motion (ROM) exercises
- ☐ Demonstration of correct use of assistive devices
- ☐ Demonstration of proper transfer techniques
- ☐ Demonstration of muscle-strengthening exercises

Key interventions

- Elevate stump for 24 hours by raising foot of bed. For upper extremity amputation, elevate stump with pillows and sling. Thereafter, keep stump flat and extended to prevent joint contracture.
- For lower-extremity amputation, assist the patient to prone position four times daily.
- Assist the patient to chair within first 12 to 24 hours after surgery.
- Assist the patient with lower-extremity amputation to get up with crutches three times daily on second postoperative day.
- Explain importance of strengthening upper body and abdominal muscles to maintain stance and balance after lower-extremity amputation.
- Teach ROM exercises for biceps, triceps, abdominal, and gluteal muscles. Encourage the patient to perform these exercises 10 times every 4 hours.

- Instruct the patient to perform adduction exercises with affected arm or leg 10 times per hour after first 24 hours.
- Administer pain medication, as prescribed, before exercise and activity.
- Instruct the patient to call for assistance when getting out of bed.
- Keep bed in low position at all times. Place call bell and personal items within the patient's reach.
- Provide trapeze bar for the patient's bed.
- Teach the patient and family appropriate transfer techniques.
- Provide instruction in how to wrap stump.
- Assist the prosthetist with prosthesis fitting.
- Consult the physical therapist for additional instructions and evaluation. Reinforce instructions given by the physical therapist.
- Consult the social services department about appropriate home care referral.

NURSING DIAGNOSIS

Body image disturbance related to limb loss

DESIRED PATIENT OUTCOME

The patient will adapt to changes in body image

Outcome measurement criteria

- ☐ Verbalization of feelings about loss of limb
- ☐ Verbalization of feelings about changes in body image
- ☐ Participation in self-care activities, as tolerated
- ☐ Participation in stump care
- ☐ Viewing and touching of stump, when ready

Key interventions

- Encourage the patient to verbalize feelings about loss of limb and changes in body image.
- Create accepting atmosphere that allows the patient to grieve. Reassure the patient that feelings of grief are normal in these circumstances.
- Clarify any misconceptions the patient and family may have regarding amputation and use of prosthetic device.
- Encourage the patient to participate in self-care activities.
- Involve the patient and family in stump care early during postoperative period, if possible. However, do not force the patient to look at or touch stump.
- Introduce the patient to other persons who have adapted successfully to similar amputation.
- Provide written information to reinforce teaching provided by the physical therapist and prosthetist.
- Consult the social services department for appropriate referrals if the patient continues to have difficulty coping.

Back pain

Pain felt in the back, which may be debilitating; among the most common health problems. Back pain requiring medical management usually results from localized injury, degenerative changes, or abrupt dislocation of intervertebral disk.

NURSING DIAGNOSIS

Impaired physical mobility related to severe back pain and stringent activity restrictions

DESIRED PATIENT OUTCOME

The patient will regain pre-injury mobility level

Outcome measurement criteria

- ☐ Verbalization of adequate pain control
- ☐ Absence of complications of immobility
- ☐ Compliance with activity restrictions
- ☐ Demonstration of leg exercises
- ☐ Gradual resumption of mobility with minimal discomfort
- ☐ Correct application of back brace or corset, if applicable

Key interventions

- Assess neurologic status of legs and evaluate bowel and bladder function on admission, then daily.
- Maintain strict bed rest on a firm mattress or bed board, if ordered.
- Reposition the patient every 2 hours, using logroll technique.

- Instruct the patient not to lie prone and to keep one or both legs flexed when lying on side.
- When the patient is supine, elevate head of bed 30 to 45 degrees and flex knees 45 degrees, to decrease tension on back muscles.
- Assess each shift for complications of immobility, such as skin breakdown, atelectasis, thrombophlebitis, and constipation.
- Apply elastic stockings while the patient is on bed rest. Remove stockings for 1 hour each shift, then reapply.
- Ask the patient to describe pain, including its severity, location, and radiation.
- Explain principles of pain control, including use of muscle relaxants, nonsteroidal anti-inflammatory drugs, and analgesics.
- Apply moist heat to the patient's back for 20 minutes four times daily, as ordered.
- Teach leg exercises, including quadriceps sets, calf pumps, and ankle circles, to decrease risk of thrombophlebitis. Supervise as the patient performs each exercise 10 times, four times daily.
- Instruct the patient in correct techniques for deep breathing and using incentive spirometer.
- Encourage the patient to participate in activities to tolerance level. Evaluate amount of discomfort experienced during activity.
- Teach correct technique for applying back brace or corset, if ordered. Observe return demonstration.
- Consult the physical therapist to implement plan for progressive activity.
- Consult the dietitian to provide diet high in fiber and fluids, to help prevent constipation.

NURSING DIAGNOSIS

Altered role performance related to activity limitations and prolonged discomfort

DESIRED PATIENT OUTCOME

The patient will adapt to diminished capacity to perform usual roles during hospitalization

Outcome measurement criteria

- ☐ Verbalization of feelings about altered role performance
- ☐ Participation in planning of care and treatment
- ☐ Verbalization of support systems and resources
- ☐ Demonstration of positive coping strategies

Key interventions

- Discuss the patient's feelings about effects of back problem on role performance.
- Offer the patient as many opportunities as possible to participate in planning of care and treatment.
- Assist the patient to identify support systems, including family, friends, and clergy.
- Discuss use of healthy coping methods, such as affirmations and positive thinking, to help refocus negative feelings and promote healing.
- Be aware that the physician may order bed rest or restricted activity for up to 6 weeks, depending on severity of injury, and that many patients are not prepared psychologically or financially to endure necessary treatment.
- Consult the occupational therapist for guidance on appropriate diversional activities.

NURSING DIAGNOSIS

High risk for ineffective management of therapeutic regimen related to lack of knowledge about long-term management of back injury and pain

DESIRED PATIENT OUTCOME

The patient will demonstrate the knowledge and skills necessary to manage recovery after discharge

Outcome measurement criteria

- ☐ Adequate pain control with administration of oral medications
- ☐ Performance of activities of daily living (ADLs) independently or with minimal assistance
- ☐ Participation in physical therapy activities
- ☐ Demonstration of correct technique when performing back exercises
- ☐ Adherence to activity restrictions to help prevent injury recurrence
- ☐ Verbalization of neurologic signs and symptoms to report to the physician
- ☐ Compliance with weight reduction program, if indicated

Key interventions

- Evaluate the patient's response to pain management efforts.
- Assess the patient's ability to perform ADLs.
- Briefly describe muscle function and basic anatomy and physiology of spine, intervertebral disks, and nerves.
- Discuss common causes of lower back pain, if appropriate, including muscle spasm, obesity, trauma, and pressure on nerves, which may cause sciatic pain.

- Teach correct posture, and encourage the patient to use correct posture when walking, sitting, and standing.
- Discuss principles of body mechanics when lifting, including bending knees, keeping back straight, holding object close to body, and using leg muscles.
- Reinforce the physical therapist's instructions on back exercises. Encourage the patient to perform pelvic tilt, knee-to-chest exercises, gluteal setting exercises, and modified sit-ups, as ordered, and to increase repetitions gradually during rehabilitation. Observe return demonstrations.
- Instruct the patient to begin and end all exercise sessions by applying moist heat to back for 10 minutes, to promote muscle relaxation.
- Advise the patient against sitting for prolonged periods. Encourage position changes every 20 minutes to decrease intervertebral pressure.
- Encourage the patient to sit in firm chair with straight back for maximum support and to use footstool when sitting to keep knees higher than hips.
- Instruct the patient to avoid standing for prolonged periods, wearing shoes with heels higher than ½", making twisting or jerky movements, and lifting heavy objects.
- Discuss medication regimen, including names, purposes, dosages, administration routes, and adverse effects of prescribed medications.
- Teach the patient correct use of patient-controlled analgesia (PCA) pump, if ordered. Observe return demonstration.
- Instruct the patient to report muscle atrophy, motor or sensory loss, decreased reflexes, and persistent pain to the primary health care practitioner.
- Consult the dietitian if weight-reduction diet is indicated.

Burn injury

Injury to tissues caused by thermal, radiant, chemical, or electrical agent; may be superficial, partial-thickness, or full-thickness.

NURSING DIAGNOSIS

Impaired skin integrity related to tissue trauma and skin graft donor site

DESIRED PATIENT OUTCOME

The patient will experience adequate healing of burned tissue

Outcome measurement criteria

- ☐ Vital signs within normal ranges
- ☐ Absence of redness, swelling, bleeding, foul odor, or purulent exudate at donor graft site
- ☐ Healing of donor graft site
- ☐ Absence of wound sepsis

Key interventions

- Assess skin to evaluate healing of burns, grafts, and donor sites.
- If the patient has an autograft, immobilize graft and protect it from trauma for at least 48 hours.
- Elevate graft site to highest position possible to prevent edema.
- Maintain graft dressing to prevent graft dislodgment.
- Use splints and elastic bandages over graft sites during patient activity.

- Protect donor site from infection or trauma. Limit exercise for several days.
- Assess graft for redness, purulent exudate, increased temperature, foul odor, and blood under graft. Report any of these signs to the physician immediately.
- Observe for wound sepsis.
- Inspect skin for pressure areas. Reposition the patient frequently. Use bed cradle, as needed.
- Massage unaffected areas with lotion to prevent skin breakdown.

NURSING DIAGNOSIS

Altered protection related to inadequate primary defenses

DESIRED PATIENT OUTCOME

The patient will remain free of infection and other complications

Outcome measurement criteria

- ☐ Adequate healing of burned tissue
- ☐ Clean, dry, intact tissue surrounding wound
- ☐ Oral temperature at or below 99.0° F (37.2° C)
- ☐ White blood cell count within expected range
- ☐ Absence of signs or symptoms of sepsis

Key interventions

- Maintain isolation precautions, and use strict aseptic technique during wound care, if ordered.
- Administer tetanus toxoid, as ordered.
- Assess burn for color, size, odor, and granulation tissue. Document findings.

- Clean burn wound once or twice daily with mild soap or normal saline solution. Debride with scissors, if ordered.
- Apply topical antibiotic, as ordered. Cover full-thickness burn with gauze or stretch bandages. Leave partial-thickness burn open to air.
- Limit visitors to patient's significant other. Bar visitors with upper respiratory infections.
- Monitor for adverse drug effects, such as pain, leukopenia, electrolyte depletion, and tissue damage. Report significant findings to the physician.
- Keep the patient warm during bathing, debriding, and wound dressing, to minimize evaporative fluid loss.
- Assess for signs and symptoms of sepsis, such as increased heart or respiratory rate, temperature elevation, reduced blood pressure, decreased urine output, and mentation changes. Report significant findings to the physician immediately.

NURSING DIAGNOSIS

Impaired physical mobility related to pain, decreased strength and endurance, and prescribed restrictions in positioning

DESIRED PATIENT OUTCOME

The patient will exhibit improved mobility

Outcome measurement criteria

- ☐ Maintenance of proper body alignment
- ☐ Performance of prescribed activities
- ☐ Verbalization of increased strength and endurance
- ☐ Absence of contractures

- ☐ Maintenance of anatomic and functional positioning of arms and legs
- ☐ Demonstration of improved mobility

Key interventions

- Maintain the patient in proper body alignment. Emphasize importance of maintaining proper body position, even if it causes discomfort.
- Reposition the patient frequently to minimize discomfort.
- Follow recommendations of the occupational and physical therapists to maintain anatomic and functional ability of the patient's arms and legs.
- Perform active and passive range-of-motion exercises, as ordered, to promote circulation and prevent contractures.
- Encourage the patient to perform exercises and participate in self-care activities, as tolerated, to increase strength and endurance gradually.
- Balance activities with rest.
- Encourage the patient to ambulate as soon as appropriate.

NURSING DIAGNOSIS

Fluid volume deficit related to internal fluid shifts

DESIRED PATIENT OUTCOME

The patient will maintain an adequate fluid balance

Outcome measurement criteria

- ☐ Urine output of at least 50 ml/hour
- ☐ Adequate fluid intake
- ☐ Absence of changes in level of consciousness (LOC)

- ☐ Vital signs within normal ranges
- ☐ Weight loss of no more than 2% daily
- ☐ Serum electrolyte and hematocrit values within normal ranges
- ☐ Urine specific gravity within normal range

Key interventions

- Weigh the patient within first 3 hours after burn injury to establish baseline. Thereafter, weigh daily at same time, using same scale and with the patient wearing similar clothes, for most accurate indication of fluid balance.
- Provide prescribed fluid replacement. Administer crystalloid fluids during first 24 hours, as prescribed, to replace vascular fluids that have leaked into interstitial tissue. After 24 to 48 hours, administer colloid and dextrose solutions, as prescribed, to replace colloids and evaporative fluid loss.
- Monitor fluid intake and output each shift.
- Assess LOC and vital signs at least every 4 hours, or more frequently if warranted by the patient's condition.
- Monitor serum electrolyte and hematocrit values daily, and report significant changes to the physician.
- Measure urine specific gravity every 4 hours to evaluate effectiveness of fluid replacement therapy.
- Maintain I.V. access at all times.

NURSING DIAGNOSIS

Pain related to effects of tissue destruction and exposed nerve endings

DESIRED PATIENT OUTCOME

The patient will experience a decrease in pain

Outcome measurement criteria

- ☐ Verbalization of adequate pain control
- ☐ Vital signs within normal ranges
- ☐ Tolerance of burn care and dressing changes with minimal discomfort

Key interventions

- Administer pain medication, as prescribed, 20 minutes before wound care and dressing changes.
- Administer pain medication on time and liberally, within prescribed parameters, to maintain adequate pain control.
- Use alternative pain control methods, such as guided imagery, progressive relaxation, and self-hypnosis, as adjuncts to pain medications.
- Teach the patient how to use patient-controlled analgesia pump, if appropriate. Observe return demonstration.
- Evaluate effectiveness of pain medication.
- Assess pain severity during wound care. Ask the patient to describe pain intensity on 1-to-10 scale.
- Explain all procedures thoroughly to decrease anxiety and fearful anticipation.
- Provide emotional support for the patient and family, to allay fears.
- Collaborate with the physician and clinical pharmacist if pain management is ineffective.

NURSING DIAGNOSIS

Altered nutrition: less than body requirements related to increased metabolic needs

DESIRED PATIENT OUTCOME

The patient will maintain an adequate nutritional intake

Outcome measurement criteria

- ☐ Consumption of 3,500 to 5,000 calories per day
- ☐ Serum protein and albumin levels within normal ranges
- ☐ Weight loss of no more than 2% per day, until stable
- ☐ Participation in food selection, if able

Key interventions

- Monitor serum protein and albumin levels, and report significant findings to the physician.
- Weigh the patient daily. Be aware that fluid retention causes initial weight gain, followed by rapid weight loss during diuretic phase.
- Assess bowel sounds each shift. Be aware that burn injury commonly causes paralytic ileus for 2 to 4 days.
- Provide total parenteral nutrition and hydration, as ordered, to meet the patient's nutritional needs.
- Once bowel sounds return, begin administering enteral nutrition, as ordered. Evaluate the patient's tolerance for enteral nutrition.
- When the patient can tolerate oral intake, provide meals high in calories and protein to promote healing.
- Maintain strict calorie count for each meal.
- Encourage the patient to participate in food selection.
- Suggest that the family bring the patient's favorite foods from home to enhance appetite.
- Consult the dietitian for additional instructions and evaluation of the patient's nutritional status.

NURSING DIAGNOSIS

Body image disturbance related to scarring and disfigurement

DESIRED PATIENT OUTCOME

The patient will begin the initial adjustment to changes in body image

Outcome measurement criteria

- ☐ Verbalization of concerns and fears about changes in body image
- ☐ Participation in goal-setting
- ☐ Participation in self-care activities
- ☐ Verbalization of positive statements about self
- ☐ Viewing of self in mirror, when ready

Key interventions

- Look directly at the patient when providing care. Avoid conveying rejection through words or nonverbal behavior.
- Encourage the patient to discuss concerns and feelings about burn injury, potential scarring, body image changes, and loss of function.
- Urge the patient to participate in self-care activities.
- Help the patient identify and use healthy coping strategies.
- Provide information about recovery and associated expectations.
- Encourage the patient to discuss expectations for recovery. Clarify misconceptions.
- Help the patient set realistic goals for recovery, including simple, attainable daily goals to prevent discouragement.

- Acknowledge the patient's attempts to meet goals. Celebrate successful goal completion with the patient and family.
- Encourage the patient to become involved in unit activities and to interact with other burn patients.
- Provide support when the patient views burned area for the first time.
- Provide teaching about postdischarge rehabilitation, including wound care, activity level, and use of special pressure garments to prevent scarring.
- Consult the social services department for additional evaluation and referrals.

Hip fracture

Break in integrity of hip bone structure, usually as result of fall, blow to body, or other accident. Surgical repair depends on fracture location; it most commonly involves open reduction internal fixation or hip arthroplasty to replace all or part of hip joint.

NURSING DIAGNOSIS

Pain related to effects of inflammation, surgery, and possible preexisting medical condition

DESIRED PATIENT OUTCOME

The patient will experience relief from pain

Outcome measurement criteria

- ☐ Verbalization of adequate pain control
- ☐ Vital signs within normal ranges
- ☐ Relaxed facial expression and muscle tone
- ☐ Use of relaxation techniques to reduce pain

Key interventions

- Assess for signs and symptoms of pain, including increased blood pressure, facial grimaces, shallow breathing, and restlessness.
- Explain principles of pain management, including meaning of *p.r.n.*
- Encourage the patient to request pain medication before pain becomes severe.
- Use additional pain control methods, such as relaxation, music therapy, and guided imagery, as adjuncts to pain medication.

- Administer analgesics, as prescribed, before activities.
- Discuss use of patient-controlled analgesia (PCA), if applicable. Teach the patient how to use PCA pump. Observe return demonstration.
- Reassure the patient and family that postoperative narcotic addiction is rare.
- Evaluate effectiveness of pain medication. Monitor for adverse narcotic effects, especially respiratory depression.
- Switch to oral analgesics as pain decreases and the patient can tolerate oral intake, as appropriate.
- Notify the physician immediately if the patient complains of sudden onset of increased pain accompanied by hip deformity or external rotation, because this may signal dislocation of hip joint.
- Consult the physician and clinical pharmacist if pain management is ineffective.

NURSING DIAGNOSIS

High risk for infection related to tissue and bone trauma, anesthesia, and immobility

DESIRED PATIENT OUTCOME

The patient will remain free of infection during hospitalization

Outcome measurement criteria

- ☐ Oral temperature at or below 99.0° F (37.2° C)
- ☐ White blood cell (WBC) count within normal range
- ☐ Absence of erythema, purulent drainage, and tenderness at incision site
- ☐ Approximation of wound edges
- ☐ Clear lung sounds

Key interventions

- Measure oral temperature at least every 4 hours.
- Monitor WBC count for increases that suggest infection, and report these to the physician.
- Auscultate breath sounds each shift for signs of atelectasis.
- Assess wound each shift for warmth, redness, drainage, tenderness, and odor.
- Use aseptic technique during dressing changes and wound care.
- Maintain suction on drainage device, as ordered, and monitor amount of drainage.
- Teach the patient correct techniques for deep breathing, coughing, and using incentive spirometer, to help prevent respiratory complications. Encourage the patient to perform these exercises every 2 hours while awake.
- Consult the infection control practitioner, as needed.

NURSING DIAGNOSIS

Impaired physical mobility related to postoperative pain and activity limitations

DESIRED PATIENT OUTCOME

The patient will achieve optimal mobility within activity limitations

Outcome measurement criteria

- ☐ Normal neurovascular function
- ☐ Absence of skin breakdown, thrombophlebitis, and constipation
- ☐ Adherence to positioning restrictions
- ☐ Performance of range-of-motion exercises with unaffected arms and legs

☐ Use of assistive devices to ambulate

Key interventions

- Assess legs for color, temperature, peripheral pulses, and motor and sensory functions. Report significant findings to the physician.
- Use pillows to position legs in 30-degree abduction.
- Avoid positioning the patient on operative side, unless ordered by the physician.
- Instruct the patient to avoid hip flexion of more than 60 degrees, extreme internal or external leg rotation, and full weight bearing on operative leg. Explain that flexion may progress to 90 degrees after 10 days.
- Elevate sitting surface with pillows to maintain hip flexion within prescribed limits.
- Assist the patient with dangling legs at bedside on first postoperative day, then to pivot to chair without weight bearing.
- Examine skin for signs of breakdown, including redness, tenderness, and blisters.
- Implement measures to help prevent skin breakdown, such as providing pressure-relief mattress and repositioning the patient.
- Assess for signs and symptoms of thrombophlebitis, including calf tenderness, warmth, and positive Homans' sign.
- Apply elastic stockings while the patient is on bed rest. Remove stockings for 1 hour each shift, then reapply.
- Encourage the patient to perform active dorsiflexion, plantar flexion, quadriceps setting, and gluteal setting exercises, to promote circulation and maintain muscle tone.
- Teach the patient how to use elevated toilet seat.
- Monitor fluid intake and output.

- Provide adequate nutrition to help maintain skin integrity. Offer meals and snacks high in calories and protein, to promote wound healing.
- Assess bowel sounds each shift to evaluate bowel function.
- Encourage adequate fluid and dietary fiber intake, to maintain bowel function.
- Assist the physical therapist with walking the patient with walker, using partial weight bearing. Reinforce instructions provided by the physical therapist.

NURSING DIAGNOSIS

High risk for altered thought processes related to anesthesia, narcotics, and unfamiliar surroundings

DESIRED PATIENT OUTCOME

The patient will regain preoperative thought process patterns

Outcome measurement criteria

☐ Orientation to person, place, and time

☐ Absence of physical injury during hospitalization

☐ Absence of confusion, lethargy, and drowsiness

Key interventions

- Assess for alterations in level of consciousness and behavior.
- Observe for irritability, lethargy, drowsiness, and confusion. Notify the physician of significant findings.
- Reorient the patient, as needed.
- Place clock and calendar within the patient's sight.

- Take measures to prevent injury, such as keeping side rails up, maintaining bed in low position, keeping call bell within the patient's reach, and checking on the patient frequently.
- Stay with the patient during ambulation to prevent injury.
- Explain safety precautions to the family to allay fears.

NURSING DIAGNOSIS

High risk for impaired home maintenance management related to limited mobility and need for assistance

DESIRED PATIENT OUTCOME

The patient or family will verbalize a plan to manage the patient at home

Outcome measurement criteria

☐ Verbalization of activity guidelines and restrictions

☐ Demonstration of correct wound care technique

☐ Identification of conditions to report to the primary health care practitioner

☐ Verbalization of available community and home care resources

Key interventions

- Discuss discharge plans with the family and social services department, if applicable.
- Determine type of equipment and services that the patient will need to manage recovery at home, such as walker, elevated toilet seat, physical therapy, Meals On Wheels, and a homemaker health aide.
- Encourage the patient to obtain long-handled shoehorn and reacher to assist with activities of daily living.

- Reinforce activity restrictions, and emphasize that the patient must adhere to these for 2 to 3 months.
- Teach the patient and family correct wound care technique. Observe return demonstration.
- Review correct use of walker. Observe return demonstration.
- Instruct the patient to report fever, decreased urine output, increased soreness or pain at operative site, or decreased mobility to the primary health care practitioner.
- Teach the patient and family about need for adequate fluid intake, balanced diet, and adequate rest to promote healing.
- Review names, purposes, dosages, administration routes, and common adverse effects of all prescribed medications.
- Emphasize lifelong need for antibiotic prophylaxis before undergoing invasive procedures, including dental work, to help prevent infection of prosthesis.

Knee replacement

Surgical implantation of prosthetic knee joint, such as to treat rheumatoid arthritis, degenerative joint disease, or avascular necrosis.

NURSING DIAGNOSIS

Pain related to inflammation and surgery

DESIRED PATIENT OUTCOME

The patient will verbalize relief from pain

Outcome measurement criteria

- ☐ Verbalization of adequate pain control
- ☐ Vital signs within normal ranges
- ☐ Relaxed facial expression and muscle tone
- ☐ Demonstration of relaxation techniques to reduce pain

Key interventions

- Assess for signs and symptoms of pain, including increased blood pressure, facial grimaces, shallow breathing, and restlessness.
- Explain principles of pain management, including meaning of *p.r.n.*
- Encourage the patient to request pain medication before pain becomes severe.
- Reassure the patient and family that postoperative narcotic addiction is rare.
- Use additional pain control methods, such as relaxation, music therapy, and guided imagery, as adjuncts to pain medication.

- Discuss use of patient-controlled analgesia (PCA), if applicable. Teach the patient how to use PCA pump. Observe return demonstration.
- Switch to oral analgesics as pain decreases and the patient can tolerate oral intake, as appropriate.
- Administer analgesics, as prescribed, before activities.
- Evaluate effectiveness of pain medication. Monitor for adverse narcotic effects, especially respiratory depression.
- Apply ice packs to knee for 20 to 30 minutes before and after flexion exercises.
- Consult the physician and clinical pharmacist if pain management is ineffective.

NURSING DIAGNOSIS

High risk for infection related to immobility and tissue and bone trauma

DESIRED PATIENT OUTCOME

The patient will remain free of infection during hospitalization

Outcome measurement criteria

- ☐ Oral temperature at or below 99.0° F (37.2° C)
- ☐ White blood cell (WBC) count within normal range
- ☐ Absence of erythema, purulent drainage, and tenderness at incision site
- ☐ Approximation of wound edges
- ☐ Clear lung sounds

Key interventions

- Measure oral temperature at least every 4 hours.

- Monitor WBC count for increases that suggest infection, and report these to the physician.
- Assess wound each shift for warmth, redness, drainage, tenderness, and odor.
- Use aseptic technique during dressing changes and wound care.
- Maintain suction on drainage device, as ordered, and monitor amount of drainage.
- Monitor lung sounds each shift for signs of atelectasis.
- Teach correct techniques for deep breathing, coughing, and using incentive spirometer, to help prevent respiratory complications. Encourage the patient to perform these exercises every 2 hours while awake.
- Consult the infection control practitioner, as needed.

NURSING DIAGNOSIS

Impaired physical mobility related to severe joint pain and activity limitations

DESIRED PATIENT OUTCOME

The patient will demonstrate optimal mobility within activity limitations

Outcome measurement criteria

☐ Maintenance of proper alignment of affected limb

☐ Adherence to position restrictions

☐ Performance of range-of-motion exercises with unaffected limbs

☐ Tolerance of continuous passive motion (CPM) machine

☐ Maintenance of normal neurovascular function

- ☐ Absence of skin breakdown, thrombophlebitis, and constipation
- ☐ Demonstration of use of assistive devices to ambulate

Key interventions

- Elevate affected leg on pillows for first 48 hours. Use caution when positioning leg to avoid knee flexion or hyperextension. Maintain the patient in neutral position.
- Reposition the patient every 2 hours, from side to back to side.
- On first postoperative day, assist the patient to sit in chair with leg elevated and to participate in light weight bearing to tolerance, using appropriate assistive device.
- Starting on fifth postoperative day, have the patient perform active flexion exercises three to four times daily.
- Encourage the patient to perform active dorsiflexion, plantar flexion, and quadriceps setting exercises. After drain removal, instruct the patient to perform straight-leg-raising exercises, to promote circulation and maintain muscle tone.
- Place leg in CPM machine for passive flexion-extension exercises, as ordered. Monitor the patient's tolerance of procedure.
- Apply resting knee extension immobilizer on affected leg until the patient can demonstrate independent straight-leg raising.
- Assess legs for color, temperature, peripheral pulses, and motor and sensory functions. Report significant findings to the physician.
- Examine skin for signs of breakdown, including redness, tenderness, and blisters.

- Implement measures to help prevent skin breakdown, such as providing pressure-relief mattress, repositioning the patient, and providing adequate nutrition.
- Assess for signs and symptoms of thrombophlebitis, including calf tenderness, warmth, and positive Homans' sign.
- Apply elastic stockings while the patient is on bed rest. Remove stockings for 1 hour each shift, then reapply.
- Monitor fluid intake and output.
- Provide meals and snacks high in calories and protein, to promote wound healing.
- Assess bowel sounds each shift to evaluate bowel function.
- Encourage adequate fluid and fiber intake to maintain bowel function.

NURSING DIAGNOSIS

Knowledge deficit regarding rehabilitation

DESIRED PATIENT OUTCOME

The patient will verbalize adequate knowledge of rehabilitation and follow-up care

Outcome measurement criteria

- ☐ Adherence to weight-bearing restrictions
- ☐ Demonstration of correct use of assistive devices
- ☐ Independent performance of flexion and leg-raising exercises
- ☐ Verbalization of signs and symptoms to report to the physician
- ☐ Verbalization of understanding of prescribed medication regimen

Key interventions

- Begin teaching the patient about activity restrictions and correct use of assistive devices before surgery, if possible. Observe several return demonstrations before discharge.
- Reinforce teaching provided by the physical therapist.
- Emphasize importance of adhering to weight-bearing limitations and using assistive devices to ambulate for at least 2 months, unless ordered otherwise by the physician.
- Review names, purposes, dosages, administration routes, and common adverse effects of prescribed medications.
- Instruct the patient to continue active flexion and straight-leg-raising exercises at home.
- Encourage the patient to keep appointments for continued physical therapy after discharge.
- Advise the patient to report increased joint pain, fever, swelling, warmth, or redness to the primary health care practitioner immediately.
- Stress importance of antibiotic prophylaxis before undergoing invasive procedures, to prevent bacterial infection of prosthesis.

Laminectomy

Surgical removal of posterior arch of one or more vertebrae, performed to relieve spinal cord compression caused by such conditions as bone displaced by injury or intervertebral disk degeneration or to remove all or part of herniated, displaced disk.

NURSING DIAGNOSIS

Pain related to nerve inflammation and surgical trauma

DESIRED PATIENT OUTCOME

The patient will verbalize relief from pain

Outcome measurement criteria

☐ Verbalization of adequate pain control

☐ Vital signs within normal ranges

☐ Relaxed facial expression and muscle tone

☐ Verbalization of ability to obtain uninterrupted sleep

Key interventions

- Assess for signs and symptoms of pain, including increased blood pressure, facial grimaces, shallow breathing, and restlessness.
- Maintain bed rest and proper body alignment, as ordered, to promote comfort.
- Explain principles of pain management, including meaning of *p.r.n.*
- Reassure the patient and family that postoperative narcotic addiction is rare.

- Encourage the patient to request pain medication before pain becomes severe.
- Use additional pain control methods, such as relaxation, music therapy, and guided imagery, as adjuncts to pain medication.
- Provide transcutaneous electrical nerve stimulator and teach the patient how to use it, to aid pain relief.
- Discuss use of patient-controlled analgesia (PCA), if applicable. Teach the patient how to use PCA pump. Observe return demonstration.
- Avoid administering morphine if the patient has had cervical surgery, because of risk of respiratory depression.
- Explain that preoperative numbness or pain in affected leg will persist for some time after surgery because of nerve irritation and edema and that muscle spasms are common.
- Administer analgesics, as prescribed, before activities.
- Evaluate effectiveness of pain medication. Monitor for adverse narcotic effects, especially respiratory depression.
- Switch to oral analgesics, as appropriate, as pain diminishes and the patient can tolerate oral intake.
- Consult the physician and clinical pharmacist if pain management is ineffective.

NURSING DIAGNOSIS

High risk for infection related to surgery and reduced primary defenses

DESIRED PATIENT OUTCOME

The patient will remain free of infection during hospitalization

Outcome measurement criteria

- ☐ Oral temperature at or below 99.0° F (37.2° C)
- ☐ White blood cell (WBC) count within normal range
- ☐ Absence of erythema, purulent drainage, and tenderness at incision site
- ☐ Approximation of wound edges

Key interventions

- Measure oral temperature at least every 4 hours.
- Monitor WBC count for increases that suggest infection, and report these to the physician.
- Assess wound each shift for warmth, redness, drainage, tenderness, and odor.
- Use aseptic technique during dressing changes and wound care.
- Maintain suction on drainage device, as ordered, and monitor amount of drainage.
- Consult the infection control practitioner, as needed.

NURSING DIAGNOSIS

Ineffective breathing pattern related to anesthesia, surgical incision, and pain

DESIRED PATIENT OUTCOME

The patient will maintain an adequate breathing pattern

Outcome measurement criteria

- ☐ Respiratory rate of 12 to 20 breaths/minute
- ☐ Absence of adventitious lung sounds
- ☐ Absence of signs or symptoms of pneumonia and atelectasis

☐ Demonstration of correct techniques for coughing, deep breathing, and using incentive spirometer

Key interventions

- Measure vital signs frequently.
- Assess respiratory status every 4 hours, noting adventitious lung sounds.
- After cervical surgery, observe surgical site for edema, which may cause respiratory difficulty. Make sure dressing is not too tight.
- Observe for splinting, shallow breathing, and dyspnea.
- Teach correct techniques for deep breathing, coughing, and using incentive spirometer, to help prevent respiratory complications. Encourage the patient to perform these exercises every 2 hours while awake.
- Assist with activities of daily living and early ambulation, as appropriate.

NURSING DIAGNOSIS

Impaired physical mobility related to activity restrictions and pain

DESIRED PATIENT OUTCOME

The patient will regain optimal physical mobility

Outcome measurement criteria

☐ Normal neurovascular function

☐ Maintenance of proper body alignment

☐ Performance of range-of-motion exercises

☐ Absence of skin breakdown

☐ Absence of constipation

☐ Absence of signs and symptoms of thrombophlebitis

□ Verbalization of activity restrictions

Key interventions

- Assess legs for color, temperature, and peripheral pulses each shift if the patient has had lumbar surgery. Assess arms for color, temperature, and peripheral pulses each shift if the patient has had cervical surgery.
- Maintain the patient in proper body alignment throughout all procedures.
- Use logrolling technique during repositioning.
- Explain activity limitations, and request return explanation.
- Avoid neck flexion or hyperextension if cervical laminectomy was performed.
- Instruct the patient to ask for assistance when getting out of bed.
- Keep personal items and call bell within the patient's reach.
- Limit the patient's initial activity to sitting in chair for short periods or ambulating short distances, as ordered.
- Balance activity with rest.
- Examine skin for signs of breakdown, including redness, tenderness, and blisters.
- Implement measures to help prevent skin breakdown, such as providing pressure-relief mattress, repositioning the patient, and providing adequate nutrition.
- Assess for signs and symptoms of thrombophlebitis, such as calf tenderness, warmth, and positive Homans' sign.
- Apply elastic stockings while the patient is on bed rest. Remove stockings for 1 hour each shift, then reapply.
- Monitor fluid intake and output.

- Provide meals and snacks high in calories and protein, to promote wound healing.
- Assess bowel sounds each shift to evaluate bowel function.
- Encourage adequate fluid and dietary fiber intake, to maintain bowel function.

NURSING DIAGNOSIS

Urinary retention related to anesthesia, supine position, and pain

DESIRED PATIENT OUTCOME

The patient will regain normal urine elimination

Outcome measurement criteria

- ☐ Absence of urinary urgency, bladder fullness, and suprapubic discomfort
- ☐ Absence of bladder distention
- ☐ Voiding of sufficient amounts of urine at normal intervals
- ☐ Absence of need for intermittent bladder catheterization
- ☐ Absence of signs and symptoms of urinary tract infection
- ☐ Balanced fluid intake and output

Key interventions

- Assess for complaints of urinary urgency, bladder fullness, and suprapubic discomfort.
- Palpate bladder for distention.
- Perform measures to stimulate voiding, such as running the faucet or pouring warm water over abdomen.

- Help the patient use commode rather than bedpan, to promote complete bladder emptying.
- If the patient has not voided within 8 hours of surgery, obtain order for straight catheterization.
- Remove no more than 1,000 ml of urine during catheterization.
- After catheterization, observe for signs and symptoms of urinary tract infection, including urinary frequency, urgency, and burning. Report significant findings to the physician.
- Measure fluid intake and output each shift, and report significant imbalances to the physician.

NURSING DIAGNOSIS

Ineffective management of therapeutic regimen related to lack of knowledge about discharge instructions

DESIRED PATIENT OUTCOME

The patient will verbalize adequate knowledge to incorporate the therapeutic regimen into daily life

Outcome measurement criteria

- ☐ Verbalization of postoperative activity restrictions
- ☐ Demonstration of correct wound care technique
- ☐ Verbalization of understanding of medication regimen
- ☐ Demonstration of independent ambulation
- ☐ Participation in activities of daily living (ADLs) with minimal assistance
- ☐ Verbalization of signs and symptoms to report to the primary health care practitioner

Key interventions

- Provide verbal and written information about activity restrictions. Instruct the patient to avoid pulling, pushing, bending, lifting, twisting, climbing stairs, and sitting for prolonged periods.
- Clarify with the physician how long the patient must wait before resuming driving and sexual activity.
- Instruct the patient to use correct posture and body mechanics during all activities.
- Teach the patient to use footstool when sitting, to keep knees higher than hips.
- Emphasize importance of sleeping in side-lying position to promote comfort.
- Teach the patient and family correct wound care technique. Observe return demonstrations.
- Caution the patient to avoid tub baths until healing is complete to prevent soaking of stitches, which would predispose the patient to infection. Explain that the patient may shower and should clean incision with mild soap and warm water.
- Review names, purposes, dosages, administration routes, and common adverse effects of prescribed medications.
- Evaluate the patient's ability to ambulate safely and perform ADLs with minimal assistance.
- Reinforce instructions provided by the physical therapist.
- Advise the patient to report increased fever, incisional pain, decreased motor or sensory function, difficulty standing erect, persistent headache, drainage from incision, or loss of bowel or bladder function to the primary health care practitioner immediately.

Radical neck dissection

Surgical removal of submandibular salivary gland, sternocleidomastoid muscle, internal jugular vein, and spinal accessory nerve, usually to treat cancer of neck structures; commonly performed in conjunction with total laryngectomy.

NURSING DIAGNOSIS

Ineffective airway clearance related to edema and thick secretions

DESIRED PATIENT OUTCOME

The patient will maintain a patent airway

Outcome measurement criteria

- ☐ Patent airway
- ☐ Decreased secretions
- ☐ Absence of adventitious lung sounds
- ☐ Absence of dyspnea and cyanosis
- ☐ Demonstration of ability to expectorate secretions
- ☐ Absence of signs and symptoms of aspiration

Key interventions

- Assess lung sounds and respiratory rate and effort at least every 4 hours after immediate postoperative period. Document rhonchi, crackles, and wheezes.
- Assess wound site for increasing edema every hour for first 24 hours. Report increasing edema, choking sensation, apprehension, change in quality of respirations, or tracheal shift to the physician immediately.

- Maintain drainage device to suction, as ordered. Milk drainage tubing every 1 to 2 hours for first 24 hours, then every 4 hours, as ordered. Be aware that if milking is contraindicated, the physician may order aspiration of drainage catheter every 4 hours, using blunt needle and strict aseptic technique.
- Keep head of bed elevated 30 to 45 degrees, to promote breathing.
- Reposition the patient every 2 hours to mobilize secretions.
- Provide instructions on deep breathing, coughing, and using incentive spirometer. Encourage the patient to perform these exercises every 2 hours.
- If the patient has tracheostomy, provide humidification and oxygen, as ordered.
- Suction airway, as needed.
- Teach the patient how to expectorate secretions effectively. Observe return demonstration.
- Keep tracheostomy set and manual resuscitation bag at bedside.

NURSING DIAGNOSIS

Impaired swallowing related to surgery, muscular weakness, pain, and fear

DESIRED PATIENT OUTCOME

The patient will demonstrate adequate swallowing

Outcome measurement criteria

- ☐ Absence of coughing, choking, and other signs of aspiration
- ☐ Demonstration of correct use of oral suction equipment
- ☐ Demonstration of Heimlich maneuver by family members

- [ ] Demonstration of correct use of supraglottic swallow technique

Key interventions

- Evaluate the patient's ability to swallow saliva and control secretions.
- Observe for coughing, choking, and other signs of aspiration. Report significant findings to the physician.
- Advance diet from liquids to soft foods to solids, as tolerated and ordered. Avoid foods containing lactose, which increase phlegm production.
- Stay with the patient during meals to provide reassurance and allay fears.
- Elevate head of bed 90 degrees during meals.
- Consult with the speech therapist to teach supraglottic swallow technique, which helps to protect airway and prevent aspiration if tracheostomy is present. In this technique, normal sequence is cough, breathe, take food, swallow, cough, swallow, and breathe.
- Place food in unaffected side of the patient's mouth. Inspect mouth for retained food after the patient swallows.
- Provide ongoing praise for the patient's attempts at swallowing, and document progress. Reinforce teaching provided by the speech therapist.

NURSING DIAGNOSIS

Impaired verbal communication related to surgical removal of larynx and presence of tracheostomy

DESIRED PATIENT OUTCOME

The patient will communicate needs effectively

Outcome measurement criteria

- ☐ Use of alternative communication method
- ☐ Consistent communication of needs to staff
- ☐ Demonstration of decreased frustration when communicating
- ☐ Evidence of satisfaction with chosen communication method

Key interventions

- Before surgery, explain need to choose alternative communication method for postoperative use because electrolaryngeal device may not be used for 5 to 7 days after surgery. Encourage the patient to choose from among various communication methods, such as paper and pencil and picture board.
- Teach the patient how to use chosen communication method. Involve the family in teaching sessions whenever possible.
- After surgery, flag call system with sticker indicating that the patient cannot speak.
- Provide encouragement for attempts at communication.
- Anticipate the patient's hygiene and toileting needs.
- Speak in normal tone. Do not raise voice or shout.
- Allow plenty of time for the patient to finish writing or communicating needs before responding.
- Encourage the patient to use call bell to summon assistance, and instruct the nursing and secretarial staffs to attend to the patient's call bell promptly.
- Consult the speech therapist for additional evaluation and instruction.

NURSING DIAGNOSIS

Altered nutrition: less than body requirements related to poor appetite, impaired smell and taste, and difficulty swallowing

DESIRED PATIENT OUTCOME

The patient will consume adequate nutritional intake

Outcome measurement criteria

☐ Maintenance of or increase in body weight

☐ Consumption of prescribed caloric intake

☐ Absence of difficulty swallowing

☐ Absence of need for nasogastric (NG) tube

☐ Serum protein and albumin levels within normal ranges

Key interventions

- Document height, weight, and recent weight loss on admission to establish baseline.
- Weigh the patient two to three times per week to monitor progress.
- Consult the dietitian to plan caloric and protein requirements.
- Monitor fluid intake and output each shift.
- Maintain NG tube for feedings, as ordered, for first 10 days after surgery.
- Assure patency and proper placement of NG tube before feedings.
- Provide thorough mouth and nares care while NG tube is in place.
- Assess the patient's ability to swallow before NG tube is removed.
- Monitor nutritional intake, and assess changes in

chewing and swallowing with each meal.

- Provide mouth care and administer analgesic before meals, as ordered.
- Monitor serum protein and albumin levels. Report significant changes to the physician.

NURSING DIAGNOSIS

Pain related to inflammation and surgery

DESIRED PATIENT OUTCOME

The patient will experience relief from pain

Outcome measurement criteria

☐ Communication of adequate pain control

☐ Vital signs within normal ranges

☐ Relaxed facial expression and muscle tone

☐ Communication of ability to obtain adequate sleep

Key interventions

- Assess for signs and symptoms of pain, including increased blood pressure, facial grimaces, shallow breathing, and restlessness.
- Maintain bed rest and proper body alignment to promote comfort.
- Explain principles of pain management, including meaning of *p.r.n.*
- Reassure the patient and family that postoperative narcotic addiction is rare.
- Encourage the patient to request pain medication before pain becomes severe.
- Administer analgesics, as prescribed, before self-care activities, meals, and ambulation.

- Use additional pain control methods, such as relaxation, music therapy, and guided imagery, as adjuncts to pain medication.
- Discuss use of patient-controlled analgesia (PCA), if applicable. Teach the patient how to use PCA pump. Observe return demonstration.
- Switch to oral analgesics, as appropriate, as pain decreases and the patient can tolerate oral intake.
- Evaluate effectiveness of pain medication. Monitor for adverse effects of narcotics, especially respiratory depression.
- Consult with the physician and clinical pharmacist if pain management is ineffective.

NURSING DIAGNOSIS

Body image disturbance related to changes in appearance and functional abilities secondary to radical surgery

DESIRED PATIENT OUTCOME

The patient will adapt to body image changes

Outcome measurement criteria

- ☐ Communication of concerns and feelings
- ☐ Participation in self-care activities, as tolerated
- ☐ Social interaction with staff, family, and friends
- ☐ Communication of physical, emotional, intellectual, and spiritual strengths

Key interventions

- Encourage the patient to communicate concerns and feelings about cancer, surgery, and changes in appearance.
- Assist the patient to identify physical, emotional,

intellectual, and spiritual strengths.

- Encourage the patient to participate in self-care activities, and praise efforts at participation.
- Urge the patient to interact socially with staff, family, and friends.
- Assist the family in recognizing effect of the patient's limitations.
- Explain to the patient and family that depression is common response to radical neck surgery.
- Introduce the patient to persons who have adapted successfully after same type of surgery.
- Consult with the social services department regarding the patient's counseling needs.
- Provide information about support groups and local chapter of Laryngectomees.

NURSING DIAGNOSIS

High risk for ineffective management of therapeutic regimen related to lack of knowledge about care after discharge

DESIRED PATIENT OUTCOME

The patient and family will demonstrate adequate knowledge to incorporate the therapeutic regimen into daily life

Outcome measurement criteria

☐ Effective communication

☐ Communication of signs and symptoms of infection

☐ Demonstration of correct wound care technique

☐ Performance of tracheostomy or laryngectomy care independently or with minimal assistance

☐ Performance of range-of-motion (ROM) exercises

- ☐ Communication of understanding of prescribed medication regimen

Key interventions

- Assess the patient's ability to communicate needs effectively using alternative communication methods.
- Instruct the patient to report signs and symptoms of infection, such as redness, edema, warmth, pain, and purulent drainage at incision site.
- Teach the patient and family correct procedures for wound care, suctioning, and tracheostomy or laryngectomy care. Observe several return demonstrations before discharge to ensure mastery.
- Monitor the patient's shoulder droop and ability to raise hand over head. Teach the patient how to perform ROM exercises, and encourage use of shoulder-strengthening exercises.
- Instruct the patient to wear shield over stoma when bathing.
- Emphasize need to keep stoma covered at all times by wearing stoma cover, garments with high necklines, or natural-fiber scarf.
- Advise the patient to avoid smoking, persons who smoke, and persons with respiratory infections.
- Instruct the patient to cover stoma when coughing to prevent transmission of possible infection.
- Review medication regimen, including names, purposes, dosages, administration routes, and common adverse effects of prescribed medications.
- Consult the physical therapist for additional instruction and evaluation of the patient's functional abilities.
- Refer the patient and family to community support groups, such as the American Cancer Society and the Lost Cord/New Voice Club.

Acquired immunodeficiency syndrome (AIDS)

Progressive, incurable disease characterized by disruption in cell-mediated immunity, caused by human immunodeficiency virus; eventually results in development of recurrent opportunistic infections, opportunistic cancers, or other abnormalities.

NURSING DIAGNOSIS

Ineffective individual coping related to overwhelming nature of disease

DESIRED PATIENT OUTCOME

The patient will demonstrate healthy coping skills

Outcome measurement criteria

☐ Identification of stressors

☐ Verbalization of concerns and fears

☐ Demonstration of healthy coping skills

☐ Verbalization of available resources and support systems

☐ Acceptance of help from identified support persons

Key interventions

- Assess the patient for signs of anxiety.
- Demonstrate acceptance of the patient through listening, eye contact, and touch.
- Encourage the patient to discuss concerns and fears.
- Reassure the patient that grief, anger, and guilt are

normal responses to AIDS diagnosis.

- Help the patient identify stressors.
- Create atmosphere that encourages open expression of feelings.
- Provide accurate information about AIDS and its treatment to help allay fears.
- Discuss coping strategies used successfully by the patient to deal with difficult situations in past. Help the patient adapt these strategies to present situation.
- Offer praise for using successful coping strategies.
- Identify unhealthy coping strategies, such as alcohol and drug use, and discuss their effects on immune system.
- Help the patient to identify physical, psychological, intellectual, and spiritual strengths.
- Teach relaxation techniques, such as deep breathing, music therapy, progressive relaxation, and guided imagery. Encourage the patient to use these techniques to decrease anxiety.
- Help the patient identify support persons, including family, friends, and clergy. Encourage the patient to accept help from these support persons, when needed.
- Encourage the family to bring familiar objects from home to make the patient feel more comfortable.
- Provide continuity of caregivers to minimize the patient's contact with unfamiliar staff.
- Encourage the patient and family to participate in AIDS support groups.
- Refer the patient to an appropriate mental health professional for counseling, if needed.

NURSING DIAGNOSIS

Altered protection related to compromised immune status

DESIRED PATIENT OUTCOME

The patient will remain free of new opportunistic infections and complications during hospitalization

Outcome measurement criteria

- ☐ Oral temperature at or below 99.0° F (37.2° C)
- ☐ White blood cell (WBC) and neutrophil counts within acceptable ranges
- ☐ Absence of wound and skin infections
- ☐ Absence of adventitious lung sounds
- ☐ Intact oral mucous membranes

Key interventions

- Measure oral temperature every 4 hours. Observe for fever, chills, and diaphoresis.
- Monitor WBC count and differential. Notify the physician if WBC or neutrophil count rises.
- Auscultate lungs every 4 hours. Note crackles, wheezes, and decreased breath sounds, and report significant findings immediately.
- Encourage the patient to deep-breathe, cough, and use incentive spirometer every 2 hours.
- Assess neurologic status every 4 hours. Observe for changes in level of consciousness, behavior, or mobility; headache; dizziness; blurred vision; confusion; and speech difficulties. Report significant findings immediately.
- Assess skin for signs of breakdown, such as redness, pressure areas, and blisters.
- Reposition the patient every 2 hours to prevent skin breakdown. Have the patient ambulate every 2 hours, if condition permits.
- Assess oral cavity and mucous membranes for ulcers, bleeding, and white patches.

- Report sore throat, dysphagia, and voice changes to the physician immediately.
- Provide oral hygiene before and after meals.
- Implement precautions to protect the patient, such as washing hands meticulously before entering and after leaving room, barring visitors and health care providers with infections, providing only cooked food, and barring live plants and flowers.
- Instruct the patient to use soft toothbrush or swabs covered with diluted hydrogen peroxide or toothpaste. Caution the patient to avoid using lemon-glycerin swabs and commercial mouthwashes.
- Administer nystatin mouthwash, antiviral agent, or other anti-infective agent, as prescribed, if oral yeast infection occurs.
- Administer antibiotic, analgesic, antipyretic, and anti-infective agents, as prescribed. Evaluate the patient's response to therapy.
- Use strict aseptic technique when performing invasive procedures.
- Observe invasive procedure sites for signs of infection.
- Apply lubricant to the patient's lips, as needed.

NURSING DIAGNOSIS

Altered nutrition: less than body requirements related to nausea, anorexia, and effects of medication

DESIRED PATIENT OUTCOME

The patient will maintain an adequate nutritional intake

Outcome measurement criteria

☐ Consumption of adequate calories and protein

- ☐ Maintenance of stable weight appropriate for height and build
- ☐ Serum protein and albumin levels within normal ranges
- ☐ Verbalization of decrease in nausea, vomiting, and anorexia

Key interventions

- Measure height and weight on admission to establish baseline. Weigh the patient daily thereafter.
- Ask the patient to describe normal dietary habits and preferences.
- Monitor fluid intake and output each shift.
- Monitor serum protein and albumin levels. Report significant changes to the physician.
- Observe for nausea and vomiting.
- Administer antiemetics 30 to 60 minutes before meals, as prescribed. Evaluate the patient's response.
- Provide small, frequent meals high in calories and protein. Monitor the patient's tolerance.
- Encourage the family to bring the patient's favorite foods from home to enhance appetite.
- Provide vitamin supplements, as ordered.
- Keep environment free of noxious stimuli that may contribute to anorexia.
- Consult the dietitian to evaluate the patient's need for enteral or parenteral nutrition.

NURSING DIAGNOSIS

Diarrhea related to effects of GI infection or chemotherapy

DESIRED PATIENT OUTCOME

The patient will regain normal bowel habits

Outcome measurement criteria

- ☐ Decrease in frequency of diarrhea stools
- ☐ Improved stool consistency
- ☐ Absence of perianal skin excoriation
- ☐ Absence of signs and symptoms of dehydration
- ☐ Verbalization of increased comfort

Key interventions

- Assess bowel elimination pattern, including frequency, quantity, and appearance of stools. Observe stools for fat, undigested food, and frank blood.
- Monitor fluid intake and output each shift.
- Provide adequate fluids to compensate for losses caused by diarrhea.
- Check for signs and symptoms of dehydration, such as poor skin turgor; increased temperature; dry skin; and dry, cracked mucous membranes.
- Monitor vital signs for evidence of hypovolemia.
- Monitor serum electrolyte values, and report significant changes to the physician.
- Assess perianal skin for excoriation or breakdown. Provide meticulous skin care after each bowel movement.
- Use skin barrier or fecal incontinence pouch, if necessary, to protect skin.
- Administer antidiarrheal medication, as prescribed, and evaluate effectiveness.

NURSING DIAGNOSIS

Fatigue related to disease and increased demands for physical and emotional energy

DESIRED PATIENT OUTCOME

The patient will experience a decrease in fatigue

Outcome measurement criteria

- ☐ Verbalization of decreased fatigue
- ☐ Participation in self-care activities to tolerance
- ☐ Verbalization of importance of getting adequate rest
- ☐ Verbalization of feeling rested

Key interventions

- Assess the patient's ability to participate in self-care activities. Encourage and assist with participation, as needed. Observe for shortness of breath and changes in vital signs and skin color.
- Offer praise for attempts to increase activity.
- Provide rest after self-care activities, diagnostic procedures, and physical activity.
- Assess the patient's mental status, because fatigue commonly is associated with depression.
- Provide adequate nutrition and vitamin supplements to boost the patient's energy.
- Evaluate the patient's sleep and rest patterns. Implement measures to promote 3- to 4-hour periods of uninterrupted sleep.

NURSING DIAGNOSIS

High risk for injury related to weakness, adverse effects of medications, and possible dementia

DESIRED PATIENT OUTCOME

The patient will remain free of injury during hospitalization

Outcome measurement criteria

- ☐ Absence of signs and symptoms of injury
- ☐ Orientation to person, place, and time
- ☐ Adherence to safety measures

Key interventions

- Assess level of consciousness and behavior every 4 hours.
- Reorient the patient to person, place, and time, as needed.
- Explain behavioral and neurologic changes to the family to allay fears. Encourage them to help reorient the patient.
- Keep bed in low position with side rails up to help prevent injury.
- Emphasize importance of calling for assistance when getting out of bed.
- Keep personal belongings and call bell within the patient's reach.
- If the patient's vision is deteriorating, keep furniture and personal items in same place at all times to promote familiarity.
- Check on the patient frequently.
- Place clock and calendar within the patient's sight.
- Discuss daily events to help keep the patient focused.
- Maintain calm, reassuring manner.
- Use clear, direct terms and give one instruction at a time.
- Use restraints to prevent injury, as needed. Follow institutional policies regarding their use.

NURSING DIAGNOSIS

Social isolation related to stigma associated with communicable disease

DESIRED PATIENT OUTCOME

The patient will experience a decreased sense of isolation

Outcome measurement criteria

- ☐ Maintenance of previous social relationships
- ☐ Verbalization of decreased feeling of isolation
- ☐ Participation in unit activities, as tolerated
- ☐ Social interaction with staff

Key interventions

- Assess the patient's support systems, including family, friends, and clergy.
- Create environment that encourages the patient to express feelings of isolation, sadness, and rejection.
- Encourage the patient to maintain contact with others through telephone calls, letters, and visits.
- Discuss with family and friends the importance of social contact for the patient's well-being.
- Explain to the patient, family, and friends that AIDS cannot be contracted through casual contact.
- Teach visitors about universal precautions to allay fears.
- Arrange to spend time with the patient when visitors are not expected.
- Ask the family to bring photo albums, books, videotapes, and the patient's favorite music.
- Encourage the patient to participate in unit activities and interact socially with staff to decrease feelings of isolation.
- Encourage the patient to participate in support groups.

NURSING DIAGNOSIS

High risk for body image disturbance related to weight loss, skin lesions, and alopecia

DESIRED PATIENT OUTCOME

The patient will acknowledge body image changes

Outcome measurement criteria

- ☐ Verbalization of feelings about changes in appearance
- ☐ Participation in self-care activities, as tolerated
- ☐ Participation in care and treatment decisions

Key interventions

- Determine the patient's perception of body image changes.
- Encourage the patient to discuss concerns and fears about changes in appearance and body function.
- Create accepting, supportive atmosphere.
- Use direct eye contact, smiling, and touch to convey acceptance.
- Avoid conveying distaste when providing physical care or cleaning the patient after episodes of incontinence.
- Assist family and friends in adapting to changes in the patient's body image by offering factual information and by including them in the patient's care.
- Encourage the patient to participate in care and treatment decisions to promote independence.
- Praise attempts to enhance appearance and bolster self-esteem.
- Provide information on using makeup to conceal skin lesions.
- Offer advice on use of scarves, hats, and wigs to mask alopecia.

- Refer the patient and family to an appropriate mental health professional, as needed.

NURSING DIAGNOSIS

Caregiver role strain related to complex physical and emotional demands of caring for a patient with AIDS

DESIRED PATIENT OUTCOME

The caregiver will develop positive strategies for dealing with role strain

Outcome measurement criteria

- ☐ Identification of current stressors
- ☐ Verbalization of effect of role strain on daily life
- ☐ Verbalization of feelings about competing or conflicting roles
- ☐ Demonstration of positive coping skills to deal with role strain
- ☐ Verbalization of need for respite help and recreation
- ☐ Acceptance of help from family, friends, and outside agencies

Key interventions

- Encourage the caregiver to discuss feelings and concerns. Use open, nonjudgmental approach to promote rapport.
- Help the caregiver identify and acknowledge specific stressors that increase role strain.
- Discuss positive strategies used successfully by the caregiver to deal with difficult situations in past. Help the caregiver adapt these strategies to present situation.
- Discuss the caregiver's favorite diversional activities, and explore ways to incorporate these into daily routine.

- Identify areas of knowledge deficit. Provide appropriate information to help reduce role strain.
- Assist the caregiver to identify support systems, such as family, friends, AIDS organizations, religious institutions, and clergy.
- Obtain information from the social services department regarding available community resources and long-term care placement options for the patient, if necessary.

NURSING DIAGNOSIS

Ineffective management of therapeutic regimen related to disease complexity and lack of information

DESIRED PATIENT OUTCOME

The patient and family will verbalize a plan to integrate the therapeutic regimen into daily life

Outcome measurement criteria

- ☐ Verbalization of methods to prevent disease transmission
- ☐ Identification of signs and symptoms of opportunistic infection
- ☐ Verbalization of need for adequate nutrition and hydration
- ☐ Demonstration of correct techniques for skin care, oral hygiene, and range-of-motion (ROM) exercises
- ☐ Discussion of plan to balance activity and rest
- ☐ Verbalization of prescribed medication regimen
- ☐ Identification of available community resources

Key interventions

- Explain disease transmission modes to the patient and family.

- Teach correct hand-washing techniques.
- Instruct the family to dispose of the patient's waste in separate, secure bags.
- Teach the family to wash the patient's soiled linens separately in 1% bleach solution.
- Emphasize importance of disposing of needles in impervious container.
- Review principles of safer sex and use of latex condoms.
- Teach correct techniques for skin care and oral hygiene.
- Provide instruction in ROM exercises. Observe return demonstrations.
- Teach the patient to report signs and symptoms of opportunistic infections, such as fever, cough, night sweats, swollen glands, stiff neck, headache, purplish skin blotches, easy bruising, and thrush.
- Emphasize importance of keeping home clean, especially bathroom and kitchen.
- Caution the patient to avoid touching fish tanks, bird cages, and animal waste because of risk of contracting toxoplasmosis.
- Advise the patient to balance activity with rest.
- Encourage adequate nutrition and hydration to promote wellness.
- Provide information on local organizations that provide meals for AIDS patients at home.
- Review medication regimen, including names, purposes, dosages, administration routes, and common adverse effects of prescribed medications. Provide written information or medication schedule to reinforce discussion.
- Provide information about community resources, including support groups, legal representation, and buddy programs.

Anemia

Deficiency of red blood cells (RBCs) caused by blood loss, impaired RBC production, increased RBC destruction, or nutritional deficiencies.

NURSING DIAGNOSIS

Activity intolerance related to imbalance between oxygen supply and demand

DESIRED PATIENT OUTCOME

The patient will tolerate gradual increases in activity

Outcome measurement criteria

- ☐ Vital signs within acceptable ranges during activity
- ☐ Hemoglobin and hematocrit values within normal ranges
- ☐ Performance of activities of daily living (ADLs) with minimal assistance
- ☐ Absence of dyspnea, pallor, and weakness during activity
- ☐ Verbalization of importance of balancing activity with rest
- ☐ Verbalization of feeling rested

Key interventions

- Measure vital signs every 4 hours.
- Assess vital sign changes during activity. Stay alert for dyspnea, tachycardia, and palpitations. Report significant findings to the physician.

- Monitor hemoglobin and hematocrit values, and report significant findings to the physician.
- Place the patient in comfortable position if bed rest is ordered. Reposition every 2 hours.
- Provide active and passive range-of-motion exercises four times daily.
- Assist with ADLs, as needed. Encourage the patient to participate in ADLs to promote independence and well-being.
- Provide undisturbed rest periods to conserve the patient's energy.
- Involve the patient in setting goals for increasing activity.
- Reassure the patient that fatigue will diminish as therapy continues.

NURSING DIAGNOSIS

High risk for injury related to decreased cerebral oxygenation and weakness

DESIRED PATIENT OUTCOME

The patient will remain free of injury during hospitalization

Outcome measurement criteria

- ☐ Absence of signs and symptoms of injury
- ☐ Pulse oximetry values within normal ranges
- ☐ Adherence to safety measures

Key interventions

- Assess level of consciousness and behavior every 4 hours.

- Monitor pulse oximetry values, and report significant findings to the physician.
- Reorient the patient to person, place, and time, as needed.
- Place clock and calendar within the patient's sight.
- Explain behavioral and neurologic changes to the family to allay fears. Encourage them to help reorient the patient.
- Keep bed in low position with side rails up to help prevent injury.
- Place personal belongings and call bell within the patient's reach.
- Emphasize importance of calling for assistance when getting out of bed.
- Ask the family to bring nonskid slippers or shoes for the patient to wear.
- Assist the patient with dangling legs at bedside before standing.
- Provide assistance during ambulation. Monitor for dizziness and hypotension.
- Maintain calm, reassuring manner.
- Ensure warmth by providing extra covers. Avoid heating pads.
- Use restraints to prevent injury, as needed. Follow institutional policies regarding their use.

NURSING DIAGNOSIS

High risk for infection related to decreased white blood cell (WBC) count and diminished immune response

DESIRED PATIENT OUTCOME

The patient will remain free of infection throughout hospitalization

Outcome measurement criteria

- ☐ Oral temperature at or below 99.0° F (37.2° C)
- ☐ WBC count within acceptable range
- ☐ Demonstration of adequate hygiene practices
- ☐ Absence of signs and symptoms of infection

Key interventions

- Measure oral temperature every 4 hours.
- Monitor WBC count, and report significant changes to the physician.
- Explain risk of infection to the patient and family.
- Instruct the patient to avoid persons with colds or other infections.
- Request that family members or others communicate with the patient by telephone instead of visiting when ill.
- Teach the patient and family correct hygiene techniques, including handwashing.

NURSING DIAGNOSIS

Knowledge deficit regarding disease, preventive measures, and treatment

DESIRED PATIENT OUTCOME

The patient will demonstrate the knowledge and skills needed to manage care after discharge

Outcome measurement criteria

- ☐ Identification of type of anemia that the patient has
- ☐ Verbalization of preventive measures
- ☐ Selection of appropriate foods to increase intake of vitamins and iron
- ☐ Verbalization of importance of follow-up laboratory studies
- ☐ Verbalization of signs and symptoms to report
- ☐ Verbalization of prescribed medication regimen

Key interventions

- Discuss type of anemia that the patient has (iron deficiency, pernicious, aplastic, or hemolytic).
- Review principles of infection control.
- Encourage the patient to increase iron and folic acid consumption by eating seafood; organ meats; whole grains; green, leafy vegetables; asparagus; and nuts.
- Consult dietitian for instruction regarding diet high in iron and folic acid.
- Instruct the patient to take iron supplements after meals to avoid GI irritation.
- Explain that iron supplements will turn stools black.
- Advise the patient to report nausea or diarrhea to the physician.
- Emphasize that the patient must receive regular, lifelong injections of parenteral vitamin B_{12}.
- Review prescribed medications, including names, purposes, dosages, administration routes, and common adverse effects.
- Encourage the patient to increase activity gradually, as tolerated, and to balance activity with rest.
- Emphasize importance of follow-up laboratory tests to monitor progress.

Chemotherapy

Treatment of disease with chemical agents, such as to eradicate neoplasms. Cancer chemotherapy is administered to prolong life, increase remission intervals, or palliate symptoms; drugs used for cancer chemotherapy may attack all rapidly dividing cells, both normal and cancerous.

NURSING DIAGNOSIS

Altered nutrition: less than body requirements related to nausea, vomiting, and anorexia

DESIRED PATIENT OUTCOME

The patient will maintain adequate nutritional status

Outcome measurement criteria

- ☐ Maintenance of or increase in weight
- ☐ Maintenance of adequate caloric intake
- ☐ Participation in food selection
- ☐ Serum albumin and protein levels within normal ranges
- ☐ Absence of severe nausea and vomiting
- ☐ Verbalization of measures that help control nausea and vomiting
- ☐ Verbalization of need to report significant weight loss to the primary health care practitioner

Key interventions

- Obtain baseline height and weight on admission.
- Weigh the patient daily to determine progress and to monitor for fluid retention.
- Assess bowel sounds each shift.

- Monitor serum protein and albumin levels to help determine nutritional status.
- Administer antiemetics before chemotherapy and on regular schedule afterward, as prescribed, to minimize nausea and vomiting.
- Serve small, frequent meals of nutritious soft foods and fluids. Withhold foods and fluids for 4 to 6 hours before chemotherapy to decrease gastric irritation.
- Provide oral hygiene before meals, using mild mouthwash and viscous xylocaine.
- Discuss food preferences, and encourage the patient to participate in food selection.
- Encourage the family to bring the patient's favorite foods from home, within dietary restrictions.
- Encourage the family to visit during meals to enhance the patient's enjoyment.

NURSING DIAGNOSIS

Altered oral mucous membrane related to drug-induced irritation

DESIRED PATIENT OUTCOME

The patient will exhibit healing of mucous membrane lesions

Outcome measurement criteria

- ☐ Normal color and moisture of mucous membranes, lips, tongue, and gums
- ☐ Demonstration of ability to swallow
- ☐ Absence of changes in vocal quality
- ☐ Absence of mucous membrane lesions
- ☐ Verbalization of signs and symptoms of recurrence of mucous membrane lesions

Key interventions

- Assess oral mucous membranes, lips, tongue, and gums for cracks, dryness, bleeding, and lesions.
- Observe for white patches, which suggest yeast infection.
- Administer nystatin oral suspension, as prescribed, to combat infection.
- Encourage the patient to maintain good oral hygiene.
- Discourage cigarette smoking and consumption of spicy or hot foods, hard-to-chew foods, alcohol, and acidic beverages, to help prevent oral pain and discomfort.
- Apply lubricant to the patient's lips to keep them moist.
- Observe for swallowing difficulty and changes in vocal quality.
- Encourage the patient to use a swab or soft toothbrush for oral hygiene to prevent injury.
- Emphasize the importance of postponing dental work, if possible.

NURSING DIAGNOSIS

Body image disturbance related to weight loss and alopecia

DESIRED PATIENT OUTCOME

The patient will acknowledge body image changes

Outcome measurement criteria

☐ Verbalization of feelings regarding body image changes

☐ Participation in self-care activities to tolerance

☐ Demonstration of use of accessories to disguise alopecia

☐ Verbalization of positive statements about self

Key interventions

- Determine the patient's perception of body image changes.
- Create accepting, supportive atmosphere.
- Encourage the patient to discuss concerns and fears about changes in appearance and body function.
- Reassure the patient that hair will grow back after chemotherapy ends.
- Offer tourniquet or ice cap therapy to help prevent hair loss, if desired.
- Encourage the patient to wash and comb remaining hair gently to decrease hair loss.
- Provide information on use of scarves, hats, and wigs to mask alopecia.
- Offer praise for attempts to enhance appearance and bolster self-esteem.

NURSING DIAGNOSIS

High risk for infection related to immunosuppression

DESIRED PATIENT OUTCOME

The patient will remain free of infection during hospitalization

Outcome measurement criteria

☐ Oral temperature at or below 99.0° F (37.2° C)

☐ White blood cell (WBC) count within expected range

☐ Absence of signs and symptoms of respiratory infection

☐ Absence of signs and symptoms of sepsis

Key interventions

- Measure oral temperature every 4 hours.

- Monitor WBC count, and report significant findings to the physician.
- Assess lung sounds every 4 hours. Stay alert for adventitious sounds.
- Administer antibiotics, as prescribed, and evaluate effectiveness.
- Monitor for signs and symptoms of sepsis. Notify the physician immediately if these occur.
- Place the patient in private room and implement protective isolation, if necessary.
- Prohibit patient contact with visitors and staff who have infections.
- Provide meticulous skin care and daily hygiene.
- Maintain clean environment.
- Avoid invasive procedures, including catheterization and I.V. line insertion, if possible.
- Encourage the patient to consider insertion of implantable port for chemotherapy treatments.
- Provide reassurance for the patient and family if infection occurs.

NURSING DIAGNOSIS

Altered protection related to bleeding tendency

DESIRED PATIENT OUTCOME

The patient will remain free of injury during hospitalization

Outcome measurement criteria

- ☐ Absence of signs and symptoms of injury
- ☐ Absence of ecchymosis and petechiae
- ☐ Absence of bleeding from nose and gums

- ☐ Absence of blood in urine and stool
- ☐ Platelet count within expected range for condition
- ☐ Verbalization of measures to prevent injury

Key interventions

- Measure vital signs every 4 hours.
- Monitor platelet count, and report significant findings to the physician.
- Pad bed rails, if necessary.
- Assess skin for ecchymosis and petechiae, and report either sign to the physician.
- Monitor for nosebleeds. If nosebleed occurs, tilt the patient's head forward slightly and apply pressure to bridge of nose with thumb and forefinger until bleeding stops. Pack nose with gauze, if necessary.
- Observe for bleeding gums.
- Encourage the patient to use soft toothbrush or swabs for oral hygiene. If bleeding occurs, have the patient rinse mouth with normal saline solution.
- Test urine and stool for blood.
- Provide high-fiber diet and administer stool softeners and laxatives, as ordered, to help prevent constipation.
- Avoid taking rectal temperature and giving enemas, to reduce risk of rectal bleeding.
- Maintain pressure on injection sites for 5 minutes. Maintain pressure on arterial sites for 10 minutes.

Leukemia

Malignant disease of hematopoietic system characterized by abnormal proliferation and development of leukocytes and leukocyte precursors in blood and bone marrow.

NURSING DIAGNOSIS

High risk for infection related to compromised immune system

DESIRED PATIENT OUTCOME

The patient will remain free of infection throughout hospitalization

Outcome measurement criteria

☐ Oral temperature at or below 99.0° F (37.2° C)

☐ White blood cell (WBC) count within expected range

☐ Absence of signs and symptoms of respiratory infections

☐ Absence of signs and symptoms of perirectal abscess

☐ Absence of signs and symptoms of sepsis

Key interventions

- Measure oral temperature every 4 hours.
- Monitor WBC count, and report significant findings to the physician.
- Assess lung sounds every 4 hours. Stay alert for adventitious sounds.
- Check for signs and symptoms of sepsis. Notify the physician immediately if these occur.

- Place the patient in private room. Implement protective isolation, if necessary.
- Prohibit patient contact with visitors and staff who have infections.
- Provide meticulous skin care and daily hygiene.
- Clean perianal area thoroughly after bowel movements. Inspect area for signs of abscess. Apply topical antiseptic agent, as needed.
- Maintain clean environment.
- Avoid invasive procedures, including catheterization and I.V. line insertion, if possible.
- Provide reassurance for the patient and family if infection occurs.

NURSING DIAGNOSIS

Altered protection related to decreased platelet count

DESIRED PATIENT OUTCOME

The patient will remain free of injury during hospitalization

Outcome measurement criteria

☐ Absence of signs and symptoms of injury

☐ Platelet count within expected range

☐ Absence of ecchymosis and petechiae

☐ Absence of nosebleeds

☐ Absence of blood in urine and stool

☐ Verbalization of measures to prevent injury

Key interventions

- Measure vital signs every 4 hours.

- Monitor platelet count, and report significant findings to the physician.
- Protect the patient from falls and other trauma.
- Pad bed rails, if necessary.
- Assist the patient with ambulation to prevent falls.
- Assess skin for ecchymosis or petechiae, and report either sign to the physician.
- Monitor for nosebleeds. If nosebleed occurs, tilt the patient's head forward slightly and apply pressure to bridge of nose with thumb and forefinger until bleeding stops. Pack nose with gauze, if necessary.
- Test urine and stool for blood.
- Observe for bleeding gums.
- Encourage the patient to use soft toothbrush or swabs for oral hygiene. If bleeding occurs, have the patient rinse mouth with normal saline solution.
- Avoid taking rectal temperature or giving enemas, to reduce risk of rectal bleeding.
- Maintain pressure on injection sites for 5 minutes. Maintain pressure on arterial sites for 10 minutes.

NURSING DIAGNOSIS

Decisional conflict (treatment options) related to lack of information

DESIRED PATIENT OUTCOME

The patient will make informed decisions about treatment options

Outcome measurement criteria

- ☐ Verbalization of feelings about current health status
- ☐ Identification of physical, psychological, intellectual, and spiritual strengths

- ☐ Verbalization of conflict regarding treatment options
- ☐ Discussion of consequences of various treatment options
- ☐ Participation in decisions about daily care
- ☐ Verbalization of increased comfort in making care and treatment decisions
- ☐ Acceptance of help from family, friends, and clergy

Key interventions

- Encourage the patient to discuss concerns and feelings. Provide uninterrupted time to listen.
- Acknowledge the patient's values and beliefs as well as present decisional conflict.
- Assist the patient to identify physical, psychological, intellectual, and spiritual strengths.
- Help the patient identify available treatment options.
- Provide accurate information about leukemia, chemotherapy, and bone marrow transplantation.
- Discuss possible consequences of various treatment options with the patient and family.
- Encourage and assist the patient in making decisions about daily activities, to promote autonomy and confidence in making decisions.
- Support use of religious practices and rituals during hospitalization, if the patient desires. Contact the chaplain or the patient's clergy, as requested.
- Encourage the patient to accept emotional support from family, friends, and clergy for comfort and strength.
- Demonstrate acceptance and support for the patient's decisions about treatment.

NURSING DIAGNOSIS

Fear related to uncertain course of disease and treatment

DESIRED PATIENT OUTCOME

The patient will demonstrate less fear

Outcome measurement criteria

- ☐ Verbalization of decreased fear
- ☐ Vital signs within normal ranges
- ☐ Relaxed facial expression and muscle tone
- ☐ Use of relaxation techniques to help control fear

Key interventions

- Assess for signs and symptoms of anxiety and fear.
- Determine source of the patient's fear by listening to concerns. Clarify any misconceptions and answer questions honestly.
- Listen for verbal cues indicating an increase or decrease in fear.
- Explain all procedures to help allay fear.
- Teach relaxation techniques, such as deep breathing, music therapy, and guided imagery.
- Maintain environment that is conducive to relaxation.

NURSING DIAGNOSIS

Knowledge deficit regarding follow-up care

DESIRED PATIENT OUTCOME

The patient will demonstrate adequate knowledge and skills regarding follow-up care

Outcome measurement criteria

- ☐ Verbalization of understanding of disease process
- ☐ Verbalization of strategies to prevent infection
- ☐ Verbalization of signs and symptoms necessitating intervention
- ☐ Identification of available community resources

Key interventions

- Explain disease process and treatments to the patient and family. Ask for return explanation to ensure comprehension.
- Review infection-prevention strategies with the patient and family.
- Advise the patient to report signs and symptoms of infection, bleeding, or fever to the primary health care practitioner.
- Discuss plan for receiving chemotherapy treatments after discharge.
- Explain importance of follow-up blood studies to monitor progress.
- Provide information about available community resources, such as the American Cancer Society and the Leukemia Society.

Lymphoma

Malignant disorder of lymphoid tissue, classified by degree and by differentiation of cell content.

NURSING DIAGNOSIS

High risk for infection related to compromised immune system

DESIRED PATIENT OUTCOME

The patient will remain free of infection throughout hospitalization

Outcome measurement criteria

- ☐ Oral temperature at or below 99.0° F (37.2° C)
- ☐ Absence of chills, flushing, and diaphoresis
- ☐ White blood cell (WBC) count within expected range
- ☐ Absence of signs and symptoms of respiratory infections
- ☐ Absence of signs and symptoms of sepsis

Key interventions

- Measure oral temperature every 4 hours.
- Monitor WBC count, and report significant findings to the physician.
- Implement comfort and cooling measures if fever is present.
- Assess lung sounds every 4 hours. Stay alert for adventitious sounds.
- Report sore throat or changes in cough, sputum, or respirations immediately.

- Monitor for complaints of urinary frequency, urgency, or burning, which may indicate urinary tract infection.
- Place the patient in private room. Implement protective isolation, if necessary.
- Prohibit patient contact with visitors and staff who have infections.
- Ensure that all visitors and staff follow strict hand-washing procedures.
- Provide meticulous skin care and daily hygiene, using mild antibacterial soap and soft cloths and towels.
- Maintain clean environment.
- Avoid invasive procedures, including catheterization and I.V. line insertion, if possible.
- Notify the physician immediately if signs or symptoms of sepsis occur.
- Provide reassurance for the patient and family if infection occurs.

NURSING DIAGNOSIS

High risk for ineffective airway clearance related to airway edema and enlarged lymph nodes

DESIRED PATIENT OUTCOME

The patient will maintain a patent airway

Outcome measurement criteria

- ☐ Clear lung sounds
- ☐ Absence of cough, hoarseness, and respiratory stridor
- ☐ Respiratory rate of 12 to 20 breaths/minute
- ☐ Demonstration of effective deep breathing and coughing
- ☐ Demonstration of ability to clear secretions from airway

Key interventions

- Assess respiratory status every 4 hours, including rate and depth of respirations, breathing pattern, and breath sounds.
- Position the patient to promote respiration and comfort, such as sitting upright.
- Encourage the patient to perform deep breathing and turning exercises every 2 hours while awake.
- Monitor for respiratory stridor, cough, and hoarseness, which indicate airway edema.
- Administer oxygen, as needed and prescribed.
- Monitor the patient's response to activity. Assist with activities to prevent respiratory distress, as necessary.
- Keep emergency airway equipment at bedside.

NURSING DIAGNOSIS

Altered nutrition: less than body requirements related to abdominal distention secondary to splenomegaly or hepatomegaly

DESIRED PATIENT OUTCOME

The patient will maintain adequate nutritional intake

Outcome measurement criteria

☐ Consumption of adequate nutritional and fluid intake

☐ Maintenance of stable weight

☐ Absence of further increase in abdominal distention

☐ Balanced fluid intake and output

Key interventions

- Assess the patient's nutritional patterns and preferences.
- Weigh the patient daily.

- Measure abdominal girth daily.
- Monitor fluid intake and output each shift.
- Provide oral hygiene before and after meals.
- Eliminate noxious stimuli that may contribute to anorexia.
- Provide small, frequent meals high in calories and protein.
- Provide high-protein liquid supplements, as needed.
- Plan rest periods before meals to conserve energy.
- Encourage the family to bring the patient's favorite foods from home and to visit during meals to enhance the patient's enjoyment.
- Have the patient sit in chair during meals, if tolerated. Encourage the patient to remain upright after meals, to decrease sensation of abdominal fullness.
- Schedule exercise between meals, if tolerated.

NURSING DIAGNOSIS

Pain related to effects of bone involvement in disease

DESIRED PATIENT OUTCOME

The patient will experience relief from pain

Outcome measurement criteria

- ☐ Verbalization of pain relief
- ☐ Vital signs within normal ranges
- ☐ Relaxed facial expression and muscle tone
- ☐ Use of relaxation techniques to control pain
- ☐ Demonstration of correct use of patient-controlled analgesic (PCA) pump, if applicable

Key interventions

- Assess pain characteristics, including severity, location, and duration.
- Explain principles of pain management, including meaning of *p.r.n.*
- Encourage the patient to request medication before pain becomes severe.
- Consider use of PCA pump if oral analgesics are ineffective.
- Teach the patient how to use PCA pump correctly. Observe return demonstration.
- Place the patient in comfortable position, maintaining correct body alignment.
- Use pillows to immobilize or support joints and extremities.
- Encourage the patient to avoid restrictive clothing that puts pressure on bones.
- Teach relaxation techniques, such as deep breathing, guided imagery, and diversion, to help control pain.
- Evaluate effectiveness of pain management.

NURSING DIAGNOSIS

Impaired skin integrity related to pruritus and immobility

DESIRED PATIENT OUTCOME

The patient will remain free of skin breakdown

Outcome measurement criteria

- ☐ Absence of evidence of skin breakdown
- ☐ Normal skin color and temperature
- ☐ Adequate skin turgor
- ☐ Absence of itching

☐ Absence of scratch marks on skin

Key interventions

- Assess skin every 4 hours for redness, pressure areas, rashes, blisters, and breaks in skin integrity.
- Keep skin moist by applying lotion.
- Reposition the patient every 2 hours.
- Encourage the patient to take oatmeal baths to soothe itching.
- Keep the patient's nails trimmed and smooth to prevent injury caused by scratching.
- Encourage the patient to apply pressure or cool cloth to itchy areas instead of scratching.
- Check the patient frequently throughout night if night sweats have been occurring. Change bed linens and provide dry gown, as needed.
- Administer medications, as prescribed, to relieve itching.
- Evaluate effectiveness of interventions to relieve itching.

NURSING DIAGNOSIS

Ineffective management of therapeutic regimen related to lack of information regarding care and treatment

DESIRED PATIENT OUTCOME

The patient and family will discuss a plan to integrate the therapeutic regimen into daily life

Outcome measurement criteria

☐ Verbalization of understanding of disease process and treatment

☐ Identification of signs and symptoms of infection and respiratory distress

- ☐ Verbalization of importance of adequate nutrition
- ☐ Verbalization of importance of balancing activity with rest
- ☐ Verbalization of prescribed medication regimen

Key interventions

- Explain disease process and treatment required after discharge.
- Encourage the patient and family to ask questions. Clarify misconceptions.
- Emphasize importance of reporting cold and flu symptoms, swallowing difficulty, fever, sore throat, urinary burning and frequency, and cuts that are slow to heal.
- Encourage the patient to avoid crowds and persons with infections.
- Teach the patient strategies to use if itching worsens.
- Instruct the patient to report early signs and symptoms of respiratory distress, such as hoarseness, cough, decreased activity tolerance, and shortness of breath.
- Explain importance of adequate nutrition, hydration, and rest.
- Encourage the patient to participate in activities of daily living, as tolerated.
- Explain need to increase activity gradually to preadmission level.
- Review medication regimen, including names, purposes, dosages, administration routes, and common adverse effects of prescribed medications.
- Discuss plans for receiving chemotherapy or radiation treatments after discharge.

Multiple myeloma

Malignant neoplasm characterized by proliferation of immature plasma cells in bone marrow, resulting in osteolytic tumors of skeleton, lymph nodes, liver, and kidney.

NURSING DIAGNOSIS

Impaired physical mobility related to effects of pathologic fractures

DESIRED PATIENT OUTCOME

The patient will attain the highest degree of mobility possible within limitations of disease

Outcome measurement criteria

- ☐ Absence of complications of immobility
- ☐ Participation in self-care activities, as tolerated
- ☐ Gradual increase in ambulation
- ☐ Absence of signs and symptoms of injury, such as from falls
- ☐ Correct use of assistive devices

Key interventions

- Assess for complications of immobility, such as pneumonia, skin breakdown, and thrombophlebitis.
- Assess reflexes, motor function, and sensation every shift. Immediately report signs and symptoms of spinal cord compression, such as sudden, severe pain and inability to move arm or leg.
- Reposition the patient carefully every 2 hours to prevent complications. Maintain proper body alignment.

- If the patient is on bed rest, promote use of trapeze bar, side rails, and footboards to assist repositioning efforts.
- Encourage deep breathing and use of incentive spirometer every 2 hours.
- Apply elastic stockings to prevent venous stasis. Remove for 1 hour each shift, then reapply.
- Consider use of pneumatic compression boots if the patient cannot tolerate elastic stockings.
- Assess the patient's ability to ambulate safely with assistive devices. Monitor gait, stance, and steadiness. Provide assistance, as needed.
- Move obstacles or furniture that could lead to bumps, falls, or other trauma.
- Keep the patient's personal items and call bell within reach.
- Provide night-light for safety.

NURSING DIAGNOSIS

Pain related to effects of bone involvement in disease

DESIRED PATIENT OUTCOME

The patient will experience relief from pain

Outcome measurement criteria

- ☐ Verbalization of pain relief
- ☐ Vital signs within normal ranges
- ☐ Relaxed facial expression and muscle tone
- ☐ Use of relaxation techniques to control pain
- ☐ Demonstration of correct use of patient-controlled analgesia (PCA) pump, if applicable

Key interventions

- Assess pain characteristics, including its severity, location, and duration.
- Explain principles of pain management, including meaning of *p.r.n.*
- Encourage the patient to request medication before pain becomes severe.
- Consider use of PCA if oral analgesics are ineffective.
- Teach the patient how to use PCA pump. Observe return demonstration.
- Place the patient in comfortable position while maintaining correct body alignment.
- Use pillows to immobilize or support joints and extremities.
- Encourage the patient to avoid restrictive clothing that puts pressure on bones.
- Use bed cradle, as needed.
- Avoid sudden movements, jarring, or other actions that might startle the patient.
- Teach the patient relaxation techniques, including deep breathing, guided imagery, and diversion, to help control pain.
- Evaluate effectiveness of pain management.

NURSING DIAGNOSIS

Altered protection related to thrombocytopenia

DESIRED PATIENT OUTCOME

The patient will remain free of injury during hospitalization

Outcome measurement criteria

- ☐ Absence of signs or symptoms of injury
- ☐ Absence of ecchymosis and petechiae
- ☐ Absence of bleeding from nose or gums
- ☐ Absence of blood in urine and stool
- ☐ Platelet count within expected range
- ☐ Verbalization of measures to prevent injury

Key interventions

- Assess vital signs every 4 hours.
- Monitor platelet count, and report significant findings to the physician.
- Pad bed rails, if necessary.
- Assess skin for ecchymosis and petechiae, and report either to the physician.
- Monitor for nosebleeds. If nosebleed occurs, tilt the patient's head forward slightly and apply pressure to bridge of nose with thumb and forefinger until bleeding stops. Pack nose with gauze, if necessary.
- Observe for bleeding from gums.
- Encourage the patient to use soft toothbrush or swabs for oral hygiene. If bleeding occurs, have the patient rinse mouth with normal saline solution.
- Test urine and stool for blood.
- Provide dietary fiber and administer stool softeners and laxatives, as ordered, to help prevent constipation.
- Avoid taking rectal temperature or giving enemas, to reduce risk of rectal bleeding.
- Maintain pressure on injection sites for 5 minutes. Maintain pressure on arterial sites for 10 minutes.

NURSING DIAGNOSIS

High risk for infection related to altered antibody formation

DESIRED PATIENT OUTCOME

The patient will remain free of infection throughout hospitalization

Outcome measurement criteria

- ☐ Oral temperature at or below 99.0° F (37.2° C)
- ☐ White blood cell (WBC) count within expected range
- ☐ Absence of signs or symptoms of respiratory infections
- ☐ Absence of signs or symptoms of sepsis

Key interventions

- Measure oral temperature every 4 hours.
- Implement comfort and cooling measures if fever is present.
- Monitor WBC count, and report significant findings to the physician.
- Assess lung sounds every 4 hours. Stay alert for adventitious sounds.
- Report sore throat or changes in cough, sputum, or respirations immediately.
- Monitor for complaints of urinary frequency, urgency, or burning, which indicate urinary tract infection.
- Check for signs or symptoms of sepsis. Notify the physician immediately if these occur.
- Place the patient in private room. Implement protective isolation, if necessary.
- Prohibit patient contact with visitors and staff who have infections.

- Make sure all visitors and staff follow strict handwashing procedures.
- Provide meticulous skin care and daily hygiene, using mild antibacterial soap and soft cloths and towels.
- Maintain clean environment.
- Avoid invasive procedures, including catheterization and I.V. line insertion, if possible.
- Provide reassurance for the patient and family if infection occurs.

NURSING DIAGNOSIS

Knowledge deficit regarding follow-up care

DESIRED PATIENT OUTCOME

The patient and family will demonstrate adequate knowledge and skills regarding follow-up care

Outcome measurement criteria

- ☐ Verbalization of understanding of disease, treatment, and prognosis
- ☐ Verbalization of strategies to prevent injury and infection
- ☐ Verbalization of pain management plan
- ☐ Demonstration of correct techniques for measuring temperature and testing urine and stool for blood
- ☐ Correct use of assistive devices
- ☐ Identification of appropriate community resources
- ☐ Verbalization of prescribed medication regimen

Key interventions

- Explain disease process and treatment required after discharge.

- Encourage the patient and family to ask questions. Clarify misconceptions.
- Emphasize importance of reporting cold and flu symptoms, fever, urinary burning and frequency, and cuts that are slow to heal.
- Encourage the patient to avoid crowds and persons with infections.
- Teach the patient to prevent skin injury by handling sharp objects carefully, using electric razors, applying sunscreen, wearing broad-brimmed hat, and avoiding going barefoot.
- Instruct the patient to avoid aspirin or aspirin-containing products unless the physician approves.
- Explain importance of adequate nutrition, hydration, and rest.
- Encourage the patient to participate in activities of daily living, as tolerated.
- Explain need to increase activity gradually to preadmission level.
- Urge the patient to avoid sports and hobbies that may cause injury.
- Review medication regimen, including names, purposes, dosages, administration routes, and common adverse effects of prescribed medications.
- Discuss plans for receiving chemotherapy or radiation treatments after discharge.

Depressive disorder

Abnormal mood state characterized by sense of worthlessness and despair, morbid thoughts, and psychomotor retardation or agitation.

NURSING DIAGNOSIS

Ineffective individual coping related to inability to express feelings

DESIRED PATIENT OUTCOME

The patient will demonstrate positive coping strategies

Outcome measurement criteria

☐ Verbalization of feelings

☐ Demonstration of increased ability to identify needs

☐ Verbalization of personal strengths

☐ Acceptance of help from others

☐ Demonstration of positive coping strategies

Key interventions

- Create atmosphere that encourages the patient to share feelings.
- Maintain nonjudgmental approach.
- Assist the patient to identify physical, psychological, intellectual, and spiritual strengths.
- Use diversional activities if the patient exhibits restlessness.

- Help the patient identify needs and communicate them to others.
- Offer encouragement for expressing needs.
- Discuss coping strategies used successfully by the patient to deal with difficult situations in past. Help the patient adapt these strategies to present situation.
- Encourage daily exercise and activity. Provide direction and assistance with activities of daily living if the patient is severely depressed.
- Teach relaxation techniques, such as deep breathing, guided imagery, music therapy, and progressive relaxation. Encourage the patient to practice such techniques several times daily.
- Help the patient identify support systems, including family members, friends, religious organizations, and clergy.
- Refer the patient to an appropriate mental health professional for ongoing counseling.

NURSING DIAGNOSIS

Altered nutrition: less than body requirements related to poor appetite and lack of interest in food

DESIRED PATIENT OUTCOME

The patient will maintain an adequate nutritional intake

Outcome measurement criteria

- ☐ Maintenance of or increase in weight
- ☐ Serum protein and albumin levels within normal ranges
- ☐ Participation in food selection
- ☐ Balanced fluid intake and output
- ☐ Verbalization of increased appetite

Key interventions

- Assess usual eating habits on admission.
- Consult the dietitian to determine the patient's caloric and protein requirements.
- Elicit the patient's food preferences. Offer preferred foods and beverages, unless contraindicated.
- Provide small, frequent meals high in calories and protein.
- Serve various food textures and tastes to stimulate the patient's appetite and interest.
- Ask the family to bring the patient's favorite foods from home.
- Encourage the family to visit during meals to enhance the patient's enjoyment.
- Offer encouragement for exhibiting increasing appetite and consuming all food served.
- Weigh the patient daily.
- Monitor serum protein and albumin levels.

NURSING DIAGNOSIS

Fatigue related to overwhelming nature of psychological demands

DESIRED PATIENT OUTCOME

The patient will experience reduced fatigue

Outcome measurement criteria

- ☐ Verbalization of reduced fatigue
- ☐ Participation in activities of daily living (ADLs), as tolerated
- ☐ Verbalization of importance of balancing activity with rest

- ☐ Participation in diversional activities
- ☐ Verbalization of feeling rested

Key interventions

- Monitor the patient for signs and symptoms of fatigue.
- Encourage participation in ADLs, as tolerated.
- Help the patient increase activity level daily to enhance well-being.
- Initiate discussion about the patient's psychological demands. Ask the patient to identify specific demands that cause fatigue and anxiety.
- Help the patient prioritize demands.
- Encourage the patient to reject additional requests and demands.
- Provide adequate rest between activities.
- Ask the patient to identify pleasurable diversional activities and encourage participation in these, to lift spirits.

NURSING DIAGNOSIS

Sleep pattern disturbance related to anxiety and worry

DESIRED PATIENT OUTCOME

The patient will demonstrate a healthy sleep pattern

Outcome measurement criteria

- ☐ Demonstration of ability to fall asleep within 20 minutes of lying down
- ☐ Performance of relaxation exercises to promote restful sleep
- ☐ Verbalization of ability to get at least 4 hours of uninterrupted sleep twice daily

□ Demonstration of decreasing episodes of excessive sleeping

Key interventions

- Assess sleeping habits to determine if the patient is getting too much or too little sleep.
- Create atmosphere conducive to sleep, such as by dimming lights, closing blinds, and eliminating interruptions and intrusions.
- Teach the patient how to use relaxation techniques, such as guided imagery, visualization, deep breathing, and progressive relaxation, to promote sleep.
- Encourage the patient to listen to soothing music, if desired.
- Instruct the patient to avoid foods and beverages containing caffeine, because these may interfere with sleep.
- Advise the patient to avoid vigorous exercise within 2 to 3 hours of retiring, because exercise has stimulant effect.
- Evaluate the patient's ability to obtain necessary rest.
- If the patient is sleeping too much, encourage regular activity and interaction with others.

NURSING DIAGNOSIS

Hopelessness related to perceived loss of control

DESIRED PATIENT OUTCOME

The patient will experience reduced feelings of hopelessness and depression

Outcome measurement criteria

□ Verbalization of sense of hope about present and future

□ Verbalization of reduced feelings of hopelessness and depression

☐ Verbalization of feeling of having regained control

☐ Absence of suicidal feelings and gestures

☐ Verbalization of importance of continuing therapy

☐ Discussion of follow-up treatment

Key interventions

- Establish trusting, supportive relationship with the patient.
- Encourage the patient to discuss feelings of hopelessness and depression.
- Assist the patient to identify positive aspects of own life and accomplishments.
- Observe the patient closely for suicidal behavior and discussion. Be aware that as mood improves, the patient may have energy to follow through on suicidal thoughts.
- Implement suicide precautions, as appropriate, according to hospital protocol.
- Once threat of suicide passes, explain need for continuing therapy after discharge.
- Review medication regimen, including names, purposes, dosages, administration routes, and common adverse effects of prescribed medications. Include the family in medication teaching.
- Encourage the patient to incorporate physical activity, adequate nutrition, and rest into daily routine.
- Ask the patient to describe plan for follow-up therapy after discharge.
- Refer the patient to an appropriate mental health professional for continued counseling.

Substance use

Use of mood-altering chemicals, such as alcohol, prescription drugs, over-the-counter preparations, or illicit drugs, that pose a potential or real threat to physical or mental health.

NURSING DIAGNOSIS

High risk for injury related to effects of withdrawal from alcohol or drugs

DESIRED PATIENT OUTCOME

The patient will remain free of injury during hospitalization

Outcome measurement criteria

☐ Absence of signs and symptoms of injury

☐ Decrease in agitation and tremors

☐ Absence of seizures

☐ Absence of hallucinations or delusions

☐ Absence of suicidal behavior

☐ Absence of evidence of alcohol or drug use

Key interventions

- Assess the patient's normal alcohol or drug use pattern. Determine type, amount, and time of last instance of alcohol or drug use.
- Monitor closely for signs and symptoms of alcohol or drug withdrawal, such as tremors, hyperactivity, agitation, increased heart and respiratory rates, increased blood pressure, disorientation, delusions, and impaired attention and memory.

- Limit number of caregivers to prevent overstimulation.
- Maintain quiet environment.
- Keep room adequately lit, especially at night, to minimize hallucinations.
- Administer sedatives, as prescribed, to prevent serious withdrawal symptoms, such as delirium tremens and seizures.
- Explain all procedures, medications, and treatments to help decrease anxiety.
- Keep bed in low position with side rails up to prevent injury.
- Apply restraints, if needed and ordered. Pad restraints to prevent skin injury. To prevent injury to the patient or staff, make sure adequate staff are available to assist with restraint application.
- Monitor the patient every 10 minutes or according to facility policy if leather restraints are used.
- Keep restraint key on hand in case of emergency.
- Release restraints one at a time to ensure adequate control of patient.
- Protect and support the patient's head and establish open airway if seizure occurs.

NURSING DIAGNOSIS

Altered nutrition: less than body requirements related to anorexia, alcohol or drug withdrawal, and lack of concern

DESIRED PATIENT OUTCOME

The patient will maintain an adequate nutritional intake

Outcome measurement criteria

☐ Maintenance of or increase in weight

- ☐ Serum protein and albumin levels within normal ranges
- ☐ Participation in food selection
- ☐ Balanced fluid intake and output
- ☐ Verbalization of increased appetite
- ☐ Consumption of all meals served

Key interventions

- Assess the patient's usual eating habits on admission.
- Consult the dietitian to determine the patient's caloric and protein requirements.
- Elicit the patient's food preferences. Offer preferred foods, unless contraindicated.
- Administer antacids and bland diet to decrease gastric discomfort.
- Provide small, frequent meals high in calories and protein. Avoid caffeinated foods and beverages.
- Serve variety of food textures and tastes to stimulate appetite and interest.
- Encourage the family to visit during meals to enhance the patient's enjoyment.
- Discuss importance of getting adequate nutrition after discharge.

NURSING DIAGNOSIS

Sleep pattern disturbance related to irritability and anxiety secondary to withdrawal

DESIRED PATIENT OUTCOME

The patient will demonstrate a healthy sleep pattern

Outcome measurement criteria

- ☐ Demonstration of ability to fall asleep within 20 minutes of lying down
- ☐ Use of relaxation exercises to promote restful sleep
- ☐ Verbalization of ability to get at least 4 hours of uninterrupted sleep twice daily
- ☐ Verbalization of feeling rested

Key interventions

- Create atmosphere conducive to sleep, such as by closing blinds and eliminating interruptions and intrusions.
- Teach the patient how to use guided imagery, visualization, deep breathing, soothing music, and progressive relaxation to promote sleep.
- Instruct the patient to avoid foods and beverages containing caffeine.
- Advise the patient to avoid vigorous exercise within 2 to 3 hours of retiring, because exercise has stimulant effect.
- Evaluate the patient's ability to obtain necessary rest.

NURSING DIAGNOSIS

Fluid volume deficit related to decreased oral intake

DESIRED PATIENT OUTCOME

The patient will demonstrate resolution of fluid volume deficit

Outcome measurement criteria

- ☐ Vital signs within normal ranges
- ☐ Serum electrolyte values within normal ranges
- ☐ Adequate fluid intake
- ☐ Balanced fluid intake and output

- ☐ Normal skin turgor
- ☐ Intact mucous membranes

Key interventions

- Monitor vital signs for evidence of hypovolemia.
- Encourage fluid intake of at least 2,500 ml/day, unless contraindicated.
- Monitor fluid intake and output each shift.
- Observe for signs and symptoms of dehydration, such as hot, dry, skin; poor skin turgor; and cracked lips and mucous membranes.
- Monitor serum electrolyte levels, and report significant findings to the physician.
- Provide preferred beverages frequently. Avoid caffeinated beverages.

NURSING DIAGNOSIS

Impaired adjustment related to denial or lack of confidence in ability to remain substance free

DESIRED PATIENT OUTCOME

The patient will acknowledge the substance abuse problem

Outcome measurement criteria

- ☐ Participation in daily group therapy sessions
- ☐ Completion of daily therapy assignments
- ☐ Verbalization of healthy coping strategies
- ☐ Incorporation of positive coping strategies into daily life
- ☐ Verbalization of commitment to remain substance free

- ☐ Verbalization of plan to participate in substance abuse program, such as Alcoholics Anonymous or Narcotics Anonymous

Key interventions

- Explain disease process of substance abuse problem.
- Assist the patient to work through denial.
- Encourage participation in daily group therapy sessions during detoxification.
- Reinforce need to take one day at a time in attempt to remain substance free.
- Help the patient identify positive coping strategies to deal with stressful situations.
- Teach the patient how to incorporate positive coping skills into daily life.
- Encourage the patient to accept support from others.
- Support the patient's commitment to remain substance free after discharge.
- Refer the patient to appropriate support groups, such as Alcoholics Anonymous or Narcotics Anonymous.
- Refer the patient's family to Al-Anon or similar support group.

NURSING DIAGNOSIS

Chronic low self-esteem related to feelings of guilt and powerlessness

DESIRED PATIENT OUTCOME

The patient will experience an increase in self-esteem

Outcome measurement criteria

- ☐ Verbalization of positive feelings about self

- ☐ Identification of personal strengths
- ☐ Verbalization of commitment to remain substance free

Key interventions

- Establish trusting relationship with the patient.
- Demonstrate caring and concern for the patient's well-being.
- Assist the patient to identify physical, psychological, intellectual, and spiritual strengths.
- Provide encouragement to build the patient's self-esteem.
- Maintain honesty and recognize need to point out the patient's manipulative behaviors, if they occur.
- Support the patient's commitment to remain substance free.
- Encourage continued therapy and participation in support group after discharge.

APPENDIX 1

NANDA taxonomy of nursing diagnoses

The currently accepted classification system for nursing diagnoses is that of the North American Nursing Diagnosis Association (NANDA), as shown in *NANDA Nursing Diagnoses: Definitions and Classification 1992-1993*. It is organized around nine human response patterns: exchanging, communicating, relating, valuing, choosing, moving, perceiving, knowing, and feeling.

The complete taxonomic structure is listed here. The series of numbers before each diagnosis is its classification number, used to determine the placement of the diagnosis within the taxonomy. The number of digits delineates the level of abstraction of the nursing diagnosis (more specific diagnoses are assigned longer numbers).

Pattern 1. Exchanging

1.1.2.1	Altered nutrition: More than body requirements
1.1.2.2	Altered nutrition: Less than body requirements
1.1.2.3	Altered nutrition: Potential for more than body requirements
1.2.1.1	High risk for infection
1.2.2.1	High risk for altered body temperature
1.2.2.2	Hypothermia
1.2.2.3	Hyperthermia
1.2.2.4	Ineffective thermoregulation
1.2.3.1	Dysreflexia
1.3.1.1	Constipation
1.3.1.1.1	Perceived constipation
1.3.1.1.2	Colonic constipation
1.3.1.2	Diarrhea
1.3.1.3	Bowel incontinence
1.3.2	Altered urinary elimination
1.3.2.1.1	Stress incontinence
1.3.2.1.2	Reflex incontinence
1.3.2.1.3	Urge incontinence
1.3.2.1.4	Functional incontinence
1.3.2.1.5	Total incontinence
1.3.2.2	Urinary retention
1.4.1.1	Altered (specify type) tissue perfusion (renal, cerebral, cardiopulmonary, gastrointestinal, peripheral)
1.4.1.2.1	Fluid volume excess
1.4.1.2.2.1	Fluid volume deficit
1.4.1.2.2.2	High risk for fluid volume deficit
1.4.2.1	Decreased cardiac output
1.5.1.1	Impaired gas exchange
1.5.1.2	Ineffective airway clearance
1.5.1.3	Ineffective breathing pattern
1.5.1.3.1	Inability to sustain spontaneous ventilation

1.5.1.3.2	Dysfunctional ventilatory weaning response
1.6.1	High risk for injury
1.6.1.1	High risk for suffocation
1.6.1.2	High risk for poisoning
1.6.1.3	High risk for trauma
1.6.1.4	High risk for aspiration
1.6.1.5	High risk for disuse syndrome
1.6.2	Altered protection
1.6.2.1	Impaired tissue integrity
1.6.2.1.1	Altered oral mucous membrane
1.6.2.1.2.1	Impaired skin integrity
1.6.2.1.2.2	High risk for impaired skin integrity

Pattern 2. Communicating

2.1.1.1	Impaired verbal communication

Pattern 3. Relating

3.1.1	Impaired social interaction
3.1.2	Social isolation
3.2.1	Altered role performance
3.2.1.1.1	Altered parenting
3.2.1.1.2	High risk for altered parenting
3.2.1.2.1	Sexual dysfunction
3.2.2	Altered family processes
3.2.2.1	Caregiver role strain
3.2.2.2	High risk for caregiver role strain
3.2.3.1	Parental role conflict
3.3	Altered sexuality patterns

Pattern 4. Valuing

4.1.1	Spiritual distress (distress of the human spirit)

Pattern 5. Choosing

5.1.1.1	Ineffective individual coping
5.1.1.1.1	Impaired adjustment
5.1.1.1.2	Defensive coping
5.1.1.1.3	Ineffective denial
5.1.2.1.1	Ineffective family coping: Disabling
5.1.2.1.2	Ineffective family coping: Compromised
5.1.2.2	Family coping: Potential for growth
5.2.1	Ineffective management of therapeutic regimen (individual)
5.2.1.1	Noncompliance (specify)
5.3.1.1	Decisional conflict (specify)
5.4	Health-seeking behaviors (specify)

Pattern 6. Moving

6.1.1.1	Impaired physical mobility
6.1.1.1.1	High risk for peripheral neurovascular dysfunction
6.1.1.2	Activity intolerance
6.1.1.2.1	Fatigue
6.1.1.3	High risk for activity intolerance
6.2.1	Sleep pattern disturbance
6.3.1.1	Diversional activity deficit
6.4.1.1	Impaired home maintenance management
6.4.2	Altered health maintenance

6.5.1	Feeding self-care deficit
6.5.1.1	Impaired swallowing
6.5.1.2	Ineffective breast-feeding
6.5.1.2.1	Interrupted breast-feeding
6.5.1.3	Effective breast-feeding
6.5.1.4	Ineffective infant feeding pattern
6.5.2	Bathing or hygiene self-care deficit
6.5.3	Dressing or grooming self-care deficit
6.5.4	Toileting self-care deficit
6.6	Altered growth and development
6.7	Relocation stress syndrome

Pattern 7. Perceiving

7.1.1	Body image disturbance
7.1.2	Self-esteem disturbance
7.1.2.1	Chronic low self-esteem
7.1.2.2	Situational low self-esteem
7.1.3	Personal identity disturbance
7.2	Sensory or perceptual alterations (specify visual, auditory, kinesthetic, gustatory, tactile, olfactory)
7.2.1.1	Unilateral neglect
7.3.1	Hopelessness
7.3.2	Powerlessness

Pattern 8. Knowing

8.1.1	Knowledge deficit (specify)
8.3	Altered thought processes

Pattern 9. Feeling

9.1.1	Pain
9.1.1.1	Chronic pain
9.2.1.1	Dysfunctional grieving
9.2.1.2	Anticipatory grieving
9.2.2	High risk for violence: Self-directed or directed at others
9.2.2.1	High risk for self-mutilation
9.2.3	Post-trauma response
9.2.3.1	Rape-trauma syndrome
9.2.3.1.1	Rape-trauma syndrome: Compound reaction
9.2.3.1.2	Rape-trauma syndrome: Silent reaction
9.3.1	Anxiety
9.3.2	Fear

APPENDIX 2

Common nursing diagnoses in medical-surgical care

The following list summarizes the nursing diagnoses that appear in this book, which are among the most common diagnoses in medical-surgical care.

Cardiovascular System

Abdominal aortic aneurysm repair
- Anxiety related to effects of impending surgical procedure and postoperative recovery
- High risk for fluid volume deficit related to complications of aneurysm repairs
- High risk for infection related to inflammation secondary to surgical trauma
- Pain related to inflammation and immobility secondary to surgical tissue trauma
- High risk for altered peripheral tissue perfusion related to reduced arterial blood flow

Acute myocardial infarction
- Activity intolerance related to imbalance between oxygen supply and demand
- Pain (chest) related to ischemia
- Ineffective denial related to perceived threat to health and lifestyle
- High risk for ineffective management of therapeutic regimen related to denial and knowledge deficit

Angina pectoris
- Pain (chest) related to imbalance between oxygen supply and demand
- Anxiety related to chest pain episodes
- High risk for altered health maintenance related to the need to modify risk factors

Cardiac arrhythmias
- High risk for decreased cardiac output related to abnormal heart rhythm
- Anxiety related to perceived threat of death

Cardiac surgery
- High risk for anxiety related to impending surgery and postoperative recovery
- Impaired physical mobility related to postoperative pain
- Ineffective breathing pattern related to incisional pain and decreased lung expansion
- High risk for infection related to inflammation secondary to surgical trauma
- High risk for ineffective management of therapeutic regimen related to required lifestyle modifications and perceived barriers to change

Congestive heart failure
- Altered cardiopulmonary tissue perfusion related to inadequate cardiac output
- Impaired gas exchange related to altered oxygen supply
- Fluid volume excess related to ventricular failure and venous congestion secondary to congestive heart failure
- Activity intolerance related to fatigue and dyspnea
- Altered nutrition: less than body requirements related to decreased appetite and dietary restrictions
- Powerlessness related to effects of chronic illness on lifestyle

Femoral-popliteal bypass
- Fear related to impending surgery and postoperative recovery
- High risk for infection related to inflammation process secondary to surgical trauma
- Pain related to inflammation process secondary to surgical tissue trauma
- High risk for peripheral neurovascular dysfunction related to reduced arterial blood flow secondary to ischemia of legs.
- Impaired physical mobility related to surgery and previous ischemic pain

Hypertension
- Pain (headache) related to increased cerebrovascular pressure secondary to hypertension
- High risk for altered cerebral tissue perfusion related to impaired circulation

- Ineffective management of therapeutic regimen related to health beliefs
- High risk for noncompliance with treatment plan related to the patient's value system

Pacemaker insertion

- Fear related to impending surgery and postoperative recovery
- High risk for decreased cardiac output related to possible pacemaker malfunction
- High risk for infection related to inflammation secondary to invasive procedure
- Pain related to inflammation secondary to surgical tissue trauma
- Altered health maintenance related to lack of knowledge regarding surgery and follow-up care

Percutaneous transluminal coronary angioplasty (PTCA)

- Fear related to lack of knowledge of procedure and perceived threat of death
- High risk for altered peripheral tissue perfusion related to possible thrombus formation secondary to PTCA
- Ineffective management of therapeutic regimen related to lack of information regarding follow-up care

Peripheral vascular disease

- Altered peripheral tissue perfusion related to reduced arterial blood flow
- Pain related to decreased circulation to extremities
- High risk for impaired skin integrity related to decreased circulation in affected extremities
- Activity intolerance related to ischemic pain

Thrombophlebitis

- Pain related to inflammation
- Altered peripheral tissue perfusion related to interruption in venous blood flow
- High risk for impaired skin integrity related to venous stasis
- High risk for impaired gas exchange related to possible embolism

- Health seeking behaviors related to prevention of recurrent thrombus formation

Respiratory System

Adult respiratory distress syndrome (ARDS)

- Impaired gas exchange related to disruption of the alveolocapillary membrane secondary to ARDS
- High risk for ineffective breathing pattern related to hypoxia and fatigue secondary to ARDS
- High risk for aspiration related to increased secretions and airway impairment
- Anxiety related to air hunger secondary to ARDS
- Ineffective individual coping related to effects of sudden onset of life-threatening condition

Asthma

- Ineffective airway clearance related to bronchospasm
- Ineffective breathing pattern related to anxiety and lung hyperinflation
- Anxiety related to difficult breathing
- High risk for infection related to steroid therapy
- Altered health maintenance related to lack of knowledge regarding preventive measures and follow-up care for asthma

Chronic airway limitation

- Ineffective airway clearance related to increased secretions and bronchospasm
- Impaired gas exchange related to airway obstruction
- Ineffective breathing pattern related to anxiety and lung hyperinflation
- Altered nutrition: less than body requirements related to shortness of breath and decreased appetite
- Sleep pattern disturbance related to stimulant effects of medication, anxiety, and shortness of breath
- Powerlessness related to effects of chronic illness on lifestyle

Lung cancer

- Pain related to inflammation process secondary to destruction of normal cells
- Altered protection related to immunosuppression secondary to chemotherapy
- Ineffective breathing pattern related to discomfort and decreased lung expansion
- Ineffective airway clearance related to bronchial obstruction secondary to tumor
- Altered nutrition: less than body requirements related to nausea, vomiting and anorexia secondary to chemotherapy
- Spiritual distress related to challenged beliefs secondary to terminal illness
- Caregiver role strain related to unpredictable course of illness

Mechanical ventilation

- Ineffective airway clearance related to intubation and copious secretions
- Ineffective breathing pattern related to neuromuscular involvement, inflammation, and decreased expansion of lungs
- High risk for infection related to stasis of secretions and loss of respiratory defenses secondary to mechanical ventilation
- Fear related to dependence on mechanical ventilator
- Impaired verbal communication related to intubation

Pneumonia

- Impaired gas exchange related to lung consolidation and increased secretions
- Ineffective airway clearance related to increased secretions
- High risk for altered body temperature related to inflammation process and invading organism
- Pain related to pleural irritation and coughing
- Ineffective management of therapeutic regimen related to lack of information about preventive measures and follow-up care

Thoracic surgery

- Fear related to impending surgery and postoperative recovery

- Pain related to inflammation secondary to surgical tissue trauma
- Ineffective breathing pattern related to pain, fatigue, and chest tubes
- High risk for infection related to surgical tissue trauma
- Impaired physical mobility related to pain, fatigue, and chest tubes

Tuberculosis

- High risk for infection transmission related to lack of knowledge and poor health practices
- Ineffective breathing pattern related to destruction of lung tissue
- Altered nutrition: less than body requirements related to fatigue and decreased appetite
- High risk for noncompliance related to complexity of treatment

Gastrointestinal System

Appendicitis

- Anxiety related to pain, impending surgery, and lack of knowledge regarding postoperative care
- Pain related to inflammation
- High risk for infection related to inflammation secondary to tissue trauma and rush of perforation

Cholecystectomy

- High risk for ineffective breathing pattern related to location of surgical incision and pain
- High risk for fluid volume deficit related to possible hemorrhage secondary to decreased vitamin K absorption
- Altered nutrition: less than body requirements related to nothing-by-mouth status, nasogastric intubation, and altered lipid metabolism
- High risk for infection related to surgical tissue trauma and drainage tubes

Cirrhosis

- Ineffective breathing pattern related to decreased lung expansion secondary to ascites
- Altered thought processes related to increased serum ammonia level secondary to liver disease
- Altered nutrition: less than body requirements related to decreased oral intake
- Fluid volume deficit related to diuretic therapy and fluid shifts secondary to liver disease
- Ineffective family coping: compromised related to progressive nature of disease
- High risk for injury related to alcohol withdrawal

Esophagitis and gastroenteritis

- Pain related to inflammation
- Altered nutrition: less than body requirements related to nausea, vomiting, and painful swallowing
- High risk for fluid volume deficit related to diarrhea and vomiting secondary to GI inflammation
- High risk for altered body temperature related to inflammation process secondary to invading organism
- Diarrhea related to invading organism

Gastrointestinal hemorrhage

- Fluid volume deficit related to blood loss
- Fatigue related to decreased oxygen supply secondary to blood loss
- Fear related to bleeding and unpredictable course of illness

Gastrointestinal surgery

- Pain related to surgery, manipulation of GI tract, and flatulence
- Ineffective breathing pattern related to narcotics and abdominal pain
- High risk for infection related to tissue trauma and increased risk of contamination secondary to intestinal surgery
- Constipation related to decreased GI motility secondary to surgery

- Impaired skin integrity related to inflammation process and excessive wound drainage
- High risk for impaired home maintenance management related to lack of information about follow-up care

Hepatitis

- Altered protection related to liver infection and invading organism
- Altered nutrition: less than body requirements related to nausea, vomiting, and anorexia
- Activity intolerance related to fatigue and weakness
- Knowledge deficit related to disease transmission and recurrence

Pancreatitis

- Altered nutrition: less than body requirements related to malabsorption
- Pain related to inflammation
- High risk for fluid volume deficit related to nausea, vomiting, and fluid shifts
- High risk for ineffective management of therapeutic regimen related to lack of information and complex nature of treatment

Ulcer disease

- Pain related to GI mucosal irritation
- High risk for fluid volume deficit related to blood loss secondary to GI hemorrhage
- Anxiety related to pain and stress
- High risk for ineffective management of therapeutic regimen related to lack of information and maladaptive coping mechanisms

Neurologic System

Cerebrovascular accident (CVA)

- Impaired physical mobility related to motor deficit secondary to CVA
- Impaired verbal communication related to damage to cerebral speech center

- High risk for impaired skin integrity related to immobility and inadequate nutrition
- Altered cerebral tissue perfusion related to interrupted arterial flow
- High risk for impaired swallowing related to neuromuscular impairment secondary to CVA
- Self-care deficit: feeding, bathing, and/or toileting related to motor deficit secondary to CVA

Intracranial surgery

- Altered cerebral tissue perfusion related to inflammation
- Pain (headache) related to craniotomy incision and possible increase in ICP
- High risk for ineffective airway clearance related to postoperative immobility and impaired cough reflex
- High risk for trauma related to altered LOC and potential for seizures secondary to increased ICP
- High risk for infection related to surgery

Meningitis

- High risk for infection related to inflammation secondary to invading organism
- High risk for altered body temperature related to inflammation process secondary to invading organism
- Pain related to inflammation
- High risk for fluid volume deficit related to fever
- Fear related to uncertainty regarding disease process

Multiple sclerosis

- High risk for ineffective airway clearance related to fatigue and muscle weakness
- Impaired physical mobility related to muscle weakness
- Self-care deficit: bathing and/or toileting related to neuromuscular impairment secondary to demyelination
- High risk for reflex incontinence related to neuromuscular impairment secondary to disease process
- High risk for bowel incontinence related to neuromuscular impairment secondary to disease process

- Altered role performance related to perception of physical limitations

Parkinson's disease
- Impaired physical mobility related to muscle weakness, rigidity, and tremors
- High risk for trauma related to unsteady gait and tremors
- Body image disturbance related to diminishing functional abilities
- High risk for caregiver role strain related to effects of neuromuscular deficits, cognitive deficits, or both

Seizure disorder
- High risk for trauma related to altered LOC and impaired autonomic function
- Anxiety related to change in health status secondary to seizure disorder
- Social isolation related to embarrassment associated with change in appearance and behavior during seizures

Spinal cord injury
- High risk for impaired skin integrity related to prolonged immobility
- Body image disturbance related to diminished motor and sensory function
- Urinary retention related to motor and sensory deficits secondary to spinal cord injury
- Bowel incontinence related to motor and sensory deficits secondary to spinal cord injury
- High risk for dysreflexia related to noxious stimuli
- Altered sexuality patterns related to motor and sensory deficits secondary to spinal cord injury

Endocrine System

Diabetes mellitus
- Altered nutrition: more than body requirements related to excessive food intake, established eating habits, and lack of information about proper nutrition

- High risk for fluid volume deficit related to excessive urinary output secondary to elevated blood glucose levels
- High risk for impaired skin integrity related to altered circulation and sensory perceptual changes
- Ineffective management of therapeutic regimen related to lack of information and complexity of required lifestyle changes

Hyperthyroidism

- High risk for altered body temperature related to increased metabolism and thyroid hormone secretion secondary to thyroid storm (hyperthyroid crisis)
- Altered nutrition: less than body requirements related to increased metabolic demand
- Ineffective individual coping related to emotional lability
- High risk for injury related to inadequate protective mechanism of eye
- High risk for ineffective management of therapeutic regimen related to lack of information about follow-up care

Hypothyroidism

- High risk for decreased cardiac output related to reduced metabolic rate
- Activity intolerance related to fatigue
- Constipation related to decreased metabolic rate
- Knowledge deficit regarding disorder, medication, regimen, and required follow-up care

Thyroidectomy

- Fear related to impending surgery and postoperative recovery
- High risk for ineffective airway clearance related to inflammation and edema secondary to surgical incision
- High risk for fluid volume deficit related to potential postoperative hemorrhage
- Pain related to inflammation process secondary to surgical tissue trauma
- Impaired verbal communication related to location of surgical incision

Genitourinary System

Acute renal failure

- Fluid volume excess related to sodium and water retention
- Altered nutrition: less than body requirements related to nausea, vomiting and dietary restrictions
- High risk for injury related to sensorimotor deficits, seizures, and bleeding secondary to nitrogenous waste retention
- High risk for infection related to diminished immune response
- Knowledge deficit regarding follow-up care necessary to prevent recurrence

Chronic renal failure

- Altered renal tissue perfusion related to irreversible kidney damage
- High risk for impaired skin integrity related to dry, itchy skin secondary to uremia
- Altered nutrition: less than body requirements related to nausea, vomiting, and anorexia
- High risk for altered thought processes related to uremia
- Powerlessness related to effects of chronic illness on lifestyle
- High risk for ineffective management of therapeutic regimen related to complex nature of disease

Hemodialysis

- High risk for fluid volume deficit related to fluid removal during dialysis and possible blood loss from access device
- High risk for infection related to invasive nature of hemodialysis
- Altered thought processes related to disequilibrium syndrome secondary to hemodialysis
- Altered family processes related to the patient's dependence on hemodialysis
- Knowledge deficit regarding dialysis and follow-up care

Nephrectomy

- High risk for fluid volume deficit related to surgery
- Pain related to location of incision

- Ineffective breathing pattern related to location of incision and narcotic analgesics
- High risk for infection related to disruption in tissue integrity
- Impaired health maintenance management related to lack of information about follow-up care

Urinary diversion
- Fear related to lack of information about surgery and presence of urinary diversion
- Altered urinary elimination related to urinary diversion
- High risk for impaired skin integrity related to urine leakage around stoma
- Body image disturbance related to presence of stoma and external pouch
- Altered health maintenance related to lack of information about urostomy

Urinary tract infection [UTI]
- Pain related to inflammation of urethra, bladder, or kidneys
- Ineffective management of therapeutic regimen related to lack of information regarding prevention of recurrent UTIs and need for follow-up care

Urolithiasis
- Pain related to spasms and anoxia of ureter wall secondary to renal calculi
- Altered urinary elimination related to pain and possible urinary tract obstruction secondary to renal calculi
- Altered health maintenance related to lack of knowledge about preventing renal calculi recurrence.

Reproductive System

Breast cancer and mastectomy
- Decisional conflict (treatment options) related to lack of information
- Fear related to uncertain course of disease and treatment
- Fluid volume excess related to impaired lymphatic drainage and surgery

- Pain related to surgery
- High risk for infection related to disruption in skin integrity and impaired lymphatic function
- Body image disturbance related to loss of breast and adverse effects of chemotherapy or radiation therapy
- Altered sexuality patterns related to perceived loss of femininity and fear of rejection
- Knowledge deficit regarding discharge instructions and follow-up care

Gynecologic surgery (major)

- Fear related to surgical outcome
- Pain related to surgical tissue trauma and manipulation of internal organs
- High risk for fluid volume deficit related to surgery
- Ineffective breathing pattern related to incisional pain and narcotic analgesics
- High risk for altered peripheral tissue perfusion related to pelvic venous stasis secondary to surgery
- High risk for infection related to surgical tissue trauma
- High risk for urinary retention related to surgical bladder manipulation
- Constipation related to decreased gastric motility secondary to narcotics and reduced oral intake
- Anticipatory grieving related to loss of reproductive capability or possible cancer diagnosis
- High risk for altered sexuality patterns related to perceived change in body image secondary to surgery
- Knowledge deficit regarding follow-up care

Penile prosthesis implantation

- Fear related to surgery and uncertain outcome
- High risk for infection related to implantation of prosthetic device
- Pain related to surgical trauma
- Situational low self-esteem related to sexual dysfunction
- Knowledge deficit regarding follow-up care

Prostate cancer

- Pain related to cancer metastasis to vertebra or spine
- Fear related to complex treatment options, altered sexuality and possibility of death prognosis
- Altered urinary elimination related to obstruction of urethra by enlarged prostate gland
- Altered protection related to immunosuppression secondary to chemotherapy or radiation therapy
- Altered nutrition: less than body requirements related to nausea, vomiting, and anorexia secondary to chemotherapy

Prostatectomy

- High risk for fluid volume deficit related to postoperative bleeding
- High risk for infection related to surgical trauma
- Pain related to bladder spasms, urinary retention and surgical trauma
- Urge incontinence related to catheter removal and changes in sphincter tone
- High risk for sexual dysfunction related to surgery
- Knowledge deficit regarding follow-up care

Testicular cancer

- Fear related to possible infertility and death secondary to cancer diagnosis
- Body image disturbance related to scrotal changes and possible breast enlargement
- Pain related to tumor or metastases to groin, retroperitoneal nodes, chest, or abdomen
- Knowledge deficit regarding postoperative care

Musculoskeletal and Integumentary Systems

Amputation

- High risk for fluid volume deficit related to postoperative hemorrhage
- High risk for infection related to disruption in skin integrity and preexisting medical condition

- Pain related to tissue, nerve, and bone trauma
- Impaired physical mobility related to loss of limb
- Body image disturbance related to limb loss

Back pain

- Impaired physical mobility related to severe back pain and stringent activity restrictions
- Altered role performance related to activity limitations and prolonged discomfort
- High risk for ineffective management of therapeutic regimen related to lack of knowledge about long-term management of back injury and pain

Burn injury

- Impaired skin integrity related to tissue trauma injury and skin graft donor site
- Altered protection related to inadequate primary defenses
- Impaired physical mobility related to pain, decreased strength and endurance, and prescribed restrictions in positioning
- Fluid volume deficit related to fluid shifts
- Pain related to tissue destruction and exposed nerve endings
- Altered nutrition: less than body requirements related to increased metabolic needs
- Body image disturbance related to scarring and disfigurement

Hip fracture

- Pain related to inflammation, surgery, and possible preexisting medication conditions
- High risk for infection related to tissue and bone trauma, anesthesia, and immobility
- Impaired physical mobility related to postoperative pain and activity limitations
- High risk for altered thought processes related to anesthesia, narcotic, and unfamiliar surroundings
- High risk for impaired home maintenance management related to limited mobility and need for assistance

Knee replacement

- Pain related to inflammation and surgery

- High risk for infection related to immobility and tissue and bone trauma
- Impaired physical mobility related to severe joint pain and activity limitations
- Knowledge deficit regarding rehabilitation

Laminectomy
- Pain related to nerve inflammation and surgical trauma
- High risk for infection related to surgery and reduced primary defenses
- Ineffective breathing patterns related to anesthesia, surgical incision, and pain
- Impaired physical mobility related to activity restrictions and pain
- Urinary retention related to anesthesia, supine position, and pain
- Ineffective management of therapeutic regimen related to lack of knowledge about discharge instructions

Radical neck dissection
- Ineffective airway clearance related to edema and thick secretions
- Impaired swallowing related to surgery, muscular weakness, pain, and fear
- Impaired verbal communication related to surgical removal of larynx and presence of tracheostomy
- Altered nutrition: less than body requirements related to poor appetite, impaired smell and taste, and difficulty swallowing
- Pain related to inflammation and surgery
- Body image disturbance related to changes in appearance and functional abilities secondary to radical surgery
- High risk for ineffective management of therapeutic regimen related to lack of knowledge about care after discharge

Hematologic and Immunologic Systems

Acquired immunodeficiency syndrome (AIDS)

- Ineffective individual coping related to overwhelming nature of disease
- Altered protection related to compromised immune status
- Altered nutrition: less than body requirements related to nausea, anorexia, and effects of medication
- Diarrhea related to GI infection or chemotherapy
- Fatigue related to disease and increased demands for physical and emotional energy
- High risk for injury related to weakness, adverse effects of medications and possible dementia
- Social isolation related to stigma associated with communicable disease
- High risk for body image disturbance related to weight loss, skin lesions, and alopecia
- Caregiver role strain related to complex physical and emotional demands of caring for a patient with AIDS
- Ineffective management of therapeutic regimen related to disease complexity and lack of information

Anemia

- Activity intolerance related to imbalance between oxygen supply and demand
- High risk for injury related to decreased cerebral oxygenation and weakness
- High risk for infection related to decreased white blood cell count and diminished immune response
- Knowledge deficit regarding disease, preventive measures, and treatment

Chemotherapy

- Altered nutrition: less than body requirements related to nausea, vomiting, and anorexia
- Altered oral mucous membrane related to drug-induced irritation
- Body image disturbance related to weight loss and alopecia

- High risk for infection related to immunosuppression
- Altered protection related to bleeding tendency

Leukemia
- High risk for infection related to compromised immune system
- Altered protection related to decreased platelet count
- Decisional conflict (treatment options) related to lack of information
- Fear related to uncertain course of disease and treatment
- Knowledge deficit regarding follow-up care

Lymphoma
- High risk for infection related to compromised immune system
- High risk for ineffective airway clearance related to airway edema and enlarged lymph nodes
- Altered nutrition: less than body requirements related to abdominal distention secondary to splenomegaly or hepatomegaly
- Pain related to bone involvement in disease
- Impaired skin integrity related to pruritus and immobility
- Ineffective management of therapeutic regimen related to lack of information regarding care and treatment

Multiple myeloma
- Impaired physical mobility related to pathologic fractures
- Pain related to effects bone involvement in disease
- Altered protection related to thrombocytopenia
- High risk for infection related to altered antibody formation
- Knowledge deficit regarding follow-up care

Psychiatric disorders

Depressive disorders
- Ineffective individual coping related to inability to express feelings

- Altered nutrition: less than body requirements related to poor appetite and lack of interest in food
- Fatigue related to overwhelming nature of psychological demands
- Sleep pattern disturbance related to anxiety and worry
- Hopelessness related to perceived loss of control

Substance use

- High risk for injury related to withdrawal effects
- Altered nutrition: less than body requirements related to anorexia, alcohol or drug withdrawal, and lack of concern
- Sleep pattern disturbance related to irritability and anxiety secondary to withdrawal
- Fluid volume deficit related to decreased oral intake
- Impaired adjustment related to denial or lack of confidence in ability to remain substance free
- Chronic low self-esteem related to feelings of guilt and powerlessness

Selected References

Books

Durham, J., and Cohen, P. (1991). *The person with AIDS: Nursing perspectives* (2nd ed.). New York: Springer Publishing.

Gordon, M. (1993). *Manual of nursing diagnosis 1993-1994.* St. Louis: Mosby-Year Book.

Holloway, N. (1993). *Medical-surgical care planning* (2nd ed.). Springhouse, PA: Springhouse Corp.

Long, B., Phipps, W., and Cassmeyer, V. (1993). *Medical-surgical nursing: A nursing process approach* (3rd ed.). St. Louis: Mosby-Year Book.

Sparks, S., and Taylor, C. (1994). *Nursing diagnosis reference manual* (3rd ed.). Springhouse, PA: Springhouse Corp.

Taptich, B., Iyer, P., and Bernocchi-Losey, D. (1994). *Nursing diagnosis and care planning* (2nd ed.). Philadelphia: W.B. Saunders Co.

Thompson, J., McFarland, G., Hirsch, J., and Tucker, S. (1993). *Mosby's clinical nursing* (3rd ed.). St. Louis: Mosby-Year Book.

Tucker, S., Canobbio, M., Paquette, E., and Wells, M. (1992). *Patient care standards: Nursing process, diagnosis, and outcome* (5th ed.). St. Louis: Mosby-Year Book.

Periodicals

Aragon, D., and Martin, M. (1993). What you should know about thrombolytic therapy for acute MI. *American Journal of Nursing,* 93(9), 24-33.

Belcaster, A. (1994). Caring for the alcohol abuser. *Nursing94,* 24(2), 56-59.

Boutotte, J. (1993). TB, the second time around. . .and how you can control it. *Nursing93,* 23(5), 42-50.

Cole-Arvin, C., Notich, L., and Underhill, A. (1994). Identifying and managing dysphagia. *Nursing94,* 24(1), 48-49.

Dunn, S. (1993). How to care for the dialysis patient. *American Journal of Nursing,* 93(6), 26-34.

Dykes, P. (1993). Minding the five P's of neurovascular assessment. *American Journal of Nursing,* 93(6), 38-39.

Flyge, H. (1993). Meeting the challenge of neutropenia. *Nursing93,* 23(7), 60-64.

Freichels, T. (1993). Orchestrating the care of mechanically ventilated patients. *American Journal of Nursing,* 93(10), 26-35.

Johannsen, J. (1993). Update: Guidelines for treating hypertension. *American Journal of Nursing,* 93(3), 42-52.

Kelly, P., and Holman, S. (1993). The new face of AIDS. *American Journal of Nursing,* 93(3), 26-36.

Laskowski-Jones, L. (1993). Acute spinal cord injury: How to minimize the damage. *American Journal of Nursing,* 93(12), 22- 32.

Macheca, M. (1993). Diabetic hypoglycemia: How to keep the threat at bay. *American Journal of Nursing,* 93(4), 26-30.

Murphy, T. (1993). Digoxin toxicity: Ventricular dysrhythmias to watch for. *American Journal of Nursing,* 93(12), 37-41.

Pellino, T. (1994). How to manage hip fractures. *American Journal of Nursing,* 94(4), 46-50.

Resnick, B. (1993). Retraining the bladder after catheterization. *American Journal of Nursing,* 93(11), 46-49.

Shantz, D., and Spitz, M. (1993). What you need to know about seizures. *Nursing93,* 23(11), 34-40.

Weilitz, P., and Dettenmeier, P. (1994). Back to basics: Test your knowledge of tracheostomy tubes. *American Journal of Nursing,* 94(2), 46-50.

Wood, L., and Gullo, S. (1993). I.V. vesicants: How to avoid extravasation with I.V. resinant drugs. *American Journal of Nursing,* 93(4), 42-46, 49-50.

Zerwekh, J. (1994). The truth-tellers: How hospice nurses help patients confront death. *American Journal of Nursing,* 94(2), 30-34.

INDEX

A

B

F

G

H

I

P